History of Medicine

It is sobering to realise that as recently as the year in which On the Origin of Species was published, learned opinion was that diseases such as typhus and cholera were spread by a 'miasma', and suggestions that doctors should wash their hands before examining patients were greeted with mockery by the profession. The Cambridge Library Collection reissues milestone publications in the history of Western medicine as well as studies of other medical traditions. Its coverage ranges from Galen on anatomical procedures to Florence Nightingale's common-sense advice to nurses, and includes early research into genetics and mental health, colonial reports on tropical diseases, documents on public health and military medicine, and publications on spa culture and medicinal plants.

The Treatment of the Insane without Mechanical Restraints

Trained as a physician and alienist (psychiatrist), John Conolly (1794–1866) first published this work in 1856. It describes the abolition of mechanical restraints in the treatment of mentally ill patients at the Hanwell County Asylum in Middlesex, where Conolly worked as resident physician. He argues for a system of non-restraint to be implemented as standard in all asylums, focusing on understanding patients as individuals and treating them with care and compassion. Conolly had introduced at Hanwell an innovative programme for patients that was based around positive activities, personal freedom, privacy, good-quality food, exercise, and, most importantly, the absence of any physical restraint. Though controversial at first, Conolly's enlightened methods and writings helped further the cause of humane treatment. This work remains a key text in the history of asylum reform and changing attitudes to mental illness.

Cambridge University Press has long been a pioneer in the reissuing of out-of-print titles from its own backlist, producing digital reprints of books that are still sought after by scholars and students but could not be reprinted economically using traditional technology. The Cambridge Library Collection extends this activity to a wider range of books which are still of importance to researchers and professionals, either for the source material they contain, or as landmarks in the history of their academic discipline.

Drawing from the world-renowned collections in the Cambridge University Library and other partner libraries, and guided by the advice of experts in each subject area, Cambridge University Press is using state-of-the-art scanning machines in its own Printing House to capture the content of each book selected for inclusion. The files are processed to give a consistently clear, crisp image, and the books finished to the high quality standard for which the Press is recognised around the world. The latest print-on-demand technology ensures that the books will remain available indefinitely, and that orders for single or multiple copies can quickly be supplied.

The Cambridge Library Collection brings back to life books of enduring scholarly value (including out-of-copyright works originally issued by other publishers) across a wide range of disciplines in the humanities and social sciences and in science and technology.

The Treatment
of the Insane
without
Mechanical Restraints

John Conolly

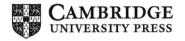
CAMBRIDGE
UNIVERSITY PRESS

CAMBRIDGE
UNIVERSITY PRESS

University Printing House, Cambridge, CB2 8BS, United Kingdom

Published in the United States of America by Cambridge University Press, New York

Cambridge University Press is part of the University of Cambridge.
It furthers the University's mission by disseminating knowledge in the pursuit of
education, learning and research at the highest international levels of excellence.

www.cambridge.org
Information on this title: www.cambridge.org/9781108063333

© in this compilation Cambridge University Press 2014

This edition first published 1856
This digitally printed version 2014

ISBN 978-1-108-06333-3 Paperback

THE TREATMENT OF THE INSANE

WITHOUT

MECHANICAL RESTRAINTS.

THE

TREATMENT OF THE INSANE

WITHOUT

MECHANICAL RESTRAINTS.

BY

JOHN CONOLLY, M.D., Edin.,

HON. D.C.L., OXON.,
FELLOW OF THE ROYAL COLLEGE OF PHYSICIANS OF LONDON,
CONSULTING PHYSICIAN TO THE MIDDLESEX LUNATIC ASYLUM AT HANWELL.

LONDON:

SMITH, ELDER & CO., 65, CORNHILL.
1856.

TO

SIR JAMES CLARK, BART., M.D., F.R.S.,

PHYSICIAN IN ORDINARY TO THE QUEEN,

AND TO

HIS ROYAL HIGHNESS PRINCE ALBERT.

MY DEAR SIR,

Chiefly by your kind encouragement, I was first induced, many years since, to compete for the office of Resident Physician in the Hanwell Asylum. In the course of the anxious labours which that appointment brought upon me, your animating approval was never wanting. My duties there being now concluded, I feel desirous, when presenting to the public a summary of the system which I endeavoured to promote, to record my deep sense of the honour of your friendship ; and, for yourself personally, my unfeigned esteem and grateful regard.

J. C.

THE LAWN HOUSE, HANWELL,
July 26*th*, 1856.

TABLE OF CONTENTS.

PART I.

THE LAST DAYS OF THE OLD METHODS OF TREATMENT.

PART II.

THE FIRST DAYS OF THE NEW OR NON-RESTRAINT SYSTEM.

PART III.

THE NEW SYSTEM IN PRIVATE ASYLUMS.

PART IV.

PART V.

PART VI.

PROGRESS OF THE NEW SYSTEM ON THE CONTINENT.

CONCLUSION.

TREATMENT OF THE INSANE,

&c., &c.

PART I.

THE LAST DAYS OF THE OLD METHODS OF TREATMENT.

WHEN the close of active professional exertions is felt to be approaching, and the pressure of that period "*aut jam urgentis aut certe adventantis senectutis*" becomes perceptible, a natural wish arises in the mind of any man who has been especially engaged in what he regards as a good and useful work to leave the work, if not finished, yet secure; or if not yet secure, at least advanced by his labours, and as little incomplete as the shortness of his life, ·and the limitation of his opportunities, permit. The accordance of such a privilege must have imposed obligations which his imperfect powers can never have fulfilled satisfactorily; and consolation under a consciousness of deficient performance can only arise from a trust in that Higher Power which allows men to be the instruments of any kind of good. Influenced by some feelings of this kind, I am anxious in these pages to explain, as distinctly as I am able, the nature, as well as the rise and progress of that method of treating the insane which is commonly called the Non-restraint System: so as to contribute to its preservation and further improvement, and perhaps to its wider adoption; or at least to prevent its being abandoned, or imperfectly acted upon, or misrepresented, when those by whom it has been steadily maintained in its early days of trial and difficulty can no longer describe or defend it.

The extent to which neglect and cruelty had reached in lunatic asylums towards the close of the last century, and which continued to prevail until a very recent period, must not be forgotten. Those who dread the accusation of a morbid philanthropy, or of visionary benevolence, may hold up in justification of their zeal the dreadful records of asylums when no pretext was given for any such accusations, and when the miserable lunatic appeared to be deserted by God and man.

Nothing, in fact, is more difficult to account for than the long neglect, in communities calling

themselves civilized, of those afflicted with a
malady so much the more dreadful than other
maladies, that before it destroys life it may be
said to destroy all that makes life valuable or
desirable. Struck with this affliction, man can no
longer enjoy the chief distinctions of his nature.
He can no longer pursue truth, nor do good, nor
govern himself. If he is a person of rank, all
his power and influence depart from him. If
he lives by the exercise of a profession, hope flies
away, and poverty overwhelms him. If he is
enterprising and speculative, prudence forsakes
him, and success crowns his enterprises no more.
If he belongs to the classes in which daily subsist-
ence is provided for by daily toil, he becomes
destitute of the means of living. No malady
effects such wide destruction, or creates so much
and such varied distress. It extinguishes knowledge; confuses eloquence, or buries it in ever-
lasting silence; it lays waste all accomplishments;
renders beauty itself painful or fearful to behold;
whilst it breaks up domestic happiness, and perverts
or annihilates all the habits and affections which
impart comfort, and joy, and value to human
existence. Yet nothing is more certain than that
this complicated misery, including every other form
of misery and mental suffering, has been, not only
the subject of neglect, but of most general abuse
and cruelty in all ages, and even down to the times

in which we live.   Knowing, as most of the readers of these observations must do, how many commodious asylums have been lately built in this country for the reception of the pauper class of the insane, they will with difficulty believe that the treatment of the maladies of the mind, or of the brain, manifesting itself in mental disorder, seems to have undergone no previous improvement, from the time of the earliest physicians whose works we possess, down to sixty years from the present day, or for about 2,500 years; and that the general management of deranged persons continued in every respect barbarous, in every country, and in every age, until Pinel in France and Tuke in England effected reforms, great in their time, often interrupted since, and even yet not universally adopted.

Up to the middle of the last century, and in many countries much later, harmless maniacs, or those supposed to be so, were allowed to wander over the country, beggars and vagabonds, affording sport and mockery. If they became troublesome, they were imprisoned in dungeons; whipped, as the phrase was, out of their madness—at all events subdued; and then secluded in darkness, in the heat of summer, and in the cold and dampness of winter, and forgotten; always half famished, often starved to death.   There was not a town or a village in all the fairest countries of Europe, nor in

all this Christian land, in which such enormities
were wholly unknown.

At length the condition of the mad obtained
some attention; and then massive and gloomy
mansions were prepared for them. These were
but prisons of the worst description. Small open-
ings in the walls, unglazed, or whether glazed or
not, guarded with strong iron bars; narrow corridors, dark cells, desolate courts, where no tree, nor
shrub, nor flower, nor blade of grass grew; solitari-
ness, or companionship so indiscriminate as to be
worse than solitude; terrible attendants, armed
with whips, sometimes (in France) accompanied by
savage dogs, and free to impose manacles, and
chains, and stripes, at their own brutal will; uncleanliness, semi-starvation, the garotte, and un-
punished murders: these were the characteristics
of such buildings throughout Europe. There were,
I need scarcely add, no gardens for exercise and
recreation, and health, such as surround all our
new asylums; no amusements, no cheerful occupations, no books to read, no newspapers or pictures,
no evening entertainments, no excursions, no animating change or variety of any kind, no scientific
medical treatment, no religious consolation. No
chapel bell assembled the patients for prayer, or
suspended the fierce and dreadful thoughts and
curses of the dungeon; no friendly face did "good
like a medicine." People looked with awe on the

outside of such buildings, and, after sunset, walked far round, to avoid hearing the cries and yells which made night hideous. Those who visited them, on some charitable mission to some not quite forgotten inmate, received impressions of terror never afterward effaced:

> Fast they found, fast shut,
> The dismal gates, and barricaded strong;
> But, long ere their approaching, heard within
> Noise, other than the sound of dance or song;
> Torment, and loud lament, and furious rage.

The recent publication of an elaborate and able Report on the General Management of the Insane of the Department, addressed by the Director of the Administration of Public Assistance to the Prefect of La Seine, including Paris, comprehends many particulars which, if not before unknown, were scattered over various publications, and scarcely available to the physician or the statesman. This report is one of three, the latest being published in 1854. All of them abound in information on every point in the management of the insane, and contain statistical tables of great interest and value.

The department of La Seine contains the large and important asylums of the Bicêtre and the Salpêtrière, to which the labours of Pinel and of Esquirol, and of their distinguished successors, Ferrus, Falret, Baillarger, Mitivié, Lélut, Trélat,

Voisin, Moreau, and others, have given the highest celebrity.*

It appears that before the period of the first great French revolution, or until the year 1790, there was no legislative protection thrown round the insane of France. In that year a law was passed to enforce the seclusion or imprisonment of the deranged and dangerous. Beyond this imperfect legislation nothing seems to have been done for nearly fifty years afterward, or until 1838, when, besides the seclusion of the insane and the mere safety of the public, the protection of their property, and the charitable care of those having no property, and the general care and comfort of persons so afflicted, first obtained public attention in that country. Attention had been given to separate the curable from those supposed to be incurable. Any arbitrary division of that kind consigns many to incurability whose recovery might be possible. But the position of the curable, who were placed in the Hôtel-Dieu, was not attended with any peculiar advantages. The wards in which they were placed were contiguous to those for patients suffering from accidents, or affected with fever ; and they slept four in a bed. The wards were narrow, and contained many rows of beds. Each ward was

* Rapport du Directeur de l'Administration de l'Assistance Publique à Monsieur le Préfet de la Seine, sur le Service des Aliénés du Département. Paris, 1852, 1853; 1854.

both a day-room and a dormitory. The treatment
of all the cases was indiscriminate. The majority
of the patients were fastened to their beds. For
the rest there were no airing courts. It is not
difficult to imagine the wretchedness and dirtiness
of such wards, and their unsuitableness to allay
mental irritation.

It would appear, from the representation of
Rochefoucault-Liancourt to the Constituent Assembly
in 1791, that the insane in England were at that
time more cared for than in France, although we
shall find that we have really little reason to boast
of our superiority at that time in this matter.

Such was the condition of the curable in the
French asylums. What, then, was the condition of
those of whose cure no hope was entertained?—
These were lodged at the Bicêtre and the
Salpêtrière; and, in both places, in cells either
attached on one side to higher terraces, or
formed below the level of the surrounding earth;
and in both cases damp and dreadful. These cells
(at the Bicêtre) were only six feet square. Air
and light were admitted by the door alone. Food
was introduced through a sort of wicket. The
only furniture consisted of narrow planks fastened
into the moist walls, and covered with straw. At
the Salpêtrière, where the cells were below the
surface, and level with the drains, large rats found
their way into them, often attacked and severely

wounded the unhappy lunatics, and sometimes occasioned their death.*

And all this existed after the luxurious age of the 14th and 15th Louis; when arts and arms, science, letters, and polished manners, made France the boast and the model of Europe.

Of the two large asylums of Paris, the Bicêtre (for men) was still the worst. In an Éloge of the famous Pinel, Dr. Pariset paints its character with his usual eloquence. The insane, the vicious, and the criminal, were mingled together, and treated alike. Wretched beings, covered with dirt, were seen crouched down in the narrow, cold, and damp cells; where scarcely air or light found way, and where there was neither table nor chair nor bench to sit upon, but only a bed of straw, very rarely renewed. The attendants on these unhappy lunatics were malefactors, selected, not for any of the gentler virtues, from the prison. The patients were loaded with chains, and defenceless against the brutality of their keepers; and the building resounded, day and night, with cries and yells, and the clanking of chains and fetters. We cannot wonder that the keepers were sometimes murdered: that the maniac, more maddened by pain and insult, often learned to dissemble his revenge, and waited to effect it.

Happily, even in the dismal period just alluded to, three enlightened and humane men were appointed

* Report to the Council of Hospitals, 1822, by M. Desportes.

administrators of the hospitals of Paris. These were Cousin, Thouret, and Cabanis. More happily still, all the three were friends of the physician PINEL; a physician whose name has become immortal. All three were of opinion that he was the only man in Paris, or even in France, who could remedy the evils which they deplored. They appointed him physician to the Bicêtre. He entered on his duties there towards the end of 1792; and with him entered, says his affectionate eulogist,* "pity, goodness, and justice." And now, slowly and cautiously, all was changed; and that amelioration commenced which, however yet imperfect and impeded, all the world acknowledges.

It is not easy to give as clear an account of the ancient state of English lunatic asylums as is afforded of those of France by the late French official reports. Long screened from public inspection, the actual condition of their inmates seems to have attracted little regard. Removed from the world, and immured in buildings on which no eye rested with pleasure, the insane were almost wholly forgotten. Everybody acknowledged that such places were repulsive in aspect, and bore a suspicious character; but it occurred to few or none of those whose thoughts were now and then turned to the probable life of the lunatics within those walls, that their condition was rendered even

* Pariset.

more dreadful by their treatment than by their malady. The affrighted visitors saw that many were furious, and it was generally admitted that severity formed a necessary part of their management; deplorable indeed, but quite essential for their proper control: and it never occurred to them that habitual severity was the real cause of the habitual fury. Before the building of what was called New Bethlem, in Moorfields, in 1675, we only read, as regards the original hospital of that name, of chains, and manacles, and the stocks. A committee, appointed in 1598, had declared the house to be so loathsome and dirty that it was not fit for any man to enter. The new building, defective as it was, became a subject of much commendation; but its praises were chiefly sung by its own officers: and we possess little authentic information as to the state of the institution, except that down to 1770 the inmates were exhibited to the public for money; that the price of admission was two-pence, and afterwards one penny.

An Act was, however, passed in 1774, for the better regulation of English madhouses, public and private, but it was extremely inefficient. Five Fellows of the College of Physicians were empowered to grant licenses for asylums, and to visit those institutions, if within seven miles of London. In the country these powers were given to justices of the peace and a physician in each county.

The powers of these visitors were nearly limited to granting licenses, which appear to have been often granted, as they still sometimes are, with as little consideration of the character of the applicant as if the license was to keep a public house. This error lies at the root of many other errors which no legislative enactments can reach or remedy, until it is remedied itself.

More than thirty years after this enactment, we are told by Dr. Haslam that lunatics, being supposed to be under the influence of the moon, were bound, chained, and even flogged at particular periods of the moon's age, to prevent the accession of violence—an atrocity almost too shocking for belief.

Indeed it would almost seem as if, at the period from the middle to near the end of the last century, the superintendents of the insane had become frantic in cruelty, from the impunity with which their despotism was attended. Some of the German physicians meditated even romantic modes of alarm and torture; wished for machinery by which a patient, just arriving at an asylum, and after being drawn with frightful clangour over a metal bridge across a moat, could be suddenly raised to the top of a tower, and as suddenly lowered into a dark and subterranean cavern; and they avowed that if the patient could be made to alight among snakes and serpents it would be better still. People not naturally cruel became habituated to severity until all feelings of humanity were forgotten. I used to be astonished, even seventeen years ago, to see humane physicians going daily round the wards of asylums, mere spectators of every form of distressing coercion, without a word of sympathy, or any order for its mitigation. But men's hearts had on this subject become gradually hardened. In medical works of authority the first principle in the treatment of lunatics was laid down to be fear, and the best means of producing fear was said to be punishment, and the best mode of punishment was defined to be stripes. The great authority of Dr. Cullen,* certainly one of the most enlightened physicians of his time, was given to this practice, although his theory of madness was that it depended upon an increased excitement of the brain.

Thus, by degrees, restraints became more and more severe, and torture more and more ingenious. Among many cruel devices, an unsuspecting patient was sometimes induced to walk across a treacherous floor ; it gave way, and the patient fell into a bath of surprise, and was there half drowned and half frightened to death.

In some continental asylums the patients were chained in a well, and the water was allowed

* First Lines of the Practice of Physic. By William Cullen, M.D., &c., &c. Part II. Book iv. (Of Mania or Madness. Sections 1559, 1564.)

gradually to ascend, in order to terrify the patient
with the prospect of inevitable death. Other
methods adopted, even within the last sixty years,
for controlling the phenomena of insanity, can
only be regarded as tacit acknowledgments of the
general inefficiency of medicine, and of the coarse
determination of vain or ignorant men to effect by
force what they could not accomplish by science.
We read with almost as much amusement as
wonder the respectful acknowledgment of Dr.
Hallaran, that Dr. Cox made known to the
profession the " safe and effectual remedy " of the
circulating swing, the invention of which Dr. Cox
" generously gives the credit of" to Dr. Darwin ;
this invention being one by means of which the
maniacal or melancholic patient, fast bound on a
sort of couch, or in a chair, was rotated at various
rates up to one hundred gyrations in a minute.
This machine was used with two indications ; the
horizontal position being adopted when the object
was to procure sleep ; and the erect posture, the
other failing in cases of excitement, to procure
intestinal action. It is acknowledged that patients
once subjected to the swing were ever afterward
terrified at the mention of it ; that it lowered the
pulse and the temperature to such a degree as to
alarm the physician ; that it occasioned a "disagree-
able suffusion of the countenance," frequently
leaving an ecchymosis of the eyes ; that it acted as

an emetic, and as a hypercathartic; but still it was lauded as reducing the unmanageable, and, stranger still, as causing the melancholy to take "a natural interest in the affairs of life." It is curious to be told, also, that the inconvenient effects mentioned were induced more certainly when the patient was in the erect position. Worse consequences occasionally resulted, I believe, from this barbarous invention; which probably rendered Dr. Hallaran's recommendation, that no "well regulated institution intended for the reception and relief of insane persons" should be unprovided with a machine of that description, ineffectual. Allusion is made to the practice in Esquirol's work (vol. i, page 156), in which he describes "la machine de Darwin" as resembling the *jeu de bague:* and he speaks of it as having passed from the arts into medicine. It found some temporary favour on the continent; but the violent evacuations produced by its employment, followed by fainting and excessive debility, led to its disuse. Dr. Cox had advised its being used in some "hopeless" cases, in the dark; with the addition of unusual noises, smells, &c.; that every sense might be assailed; but I do not think this advice was ever acted upon.

With the same simple intention of subduing violent symptoms, all the forms of mechanical restraint that ingenuity could devise seem successively to have been adopted, many of which have been from time to time reluctantly abandoned, whilst several are even now retained as essential to the control of the insane. The principal object of all such contrivances is to limit the movements of the patient, and this has been variously effected in different asylums and countries. The simplest and cheapest means was by the use of chains, to which, as more lenient, succeeded strong waistcoats confining the arms to the trunk, the legs being secured by hobbles. Handcuffs, and leather muffs and straps, have been much relied upon, with complications, in difficult cases, investing the patient with a kind of heavy circular collar and harness. Patients were seen standing by a wall to which their hands were chained, or sitting on a bench, to which they were strongly secured. Others were fastened in a sort of chair resembling the ancient watchman's box, and many were chained or strapped down in bed. The methods of restraint varied according to the ingenuity of the superintendents ; but the object of all the methods was the same—to restrain the movements of the patient. The vagrant action of the limbs was suppressed, but the source of irritation in the brain left out of consideration.

About the time when Pinel's great work of reformation was effected in France, and many patients were liberated, after being chained for many years, a similar work was providentially commenced in a provincial city in England. It began, as important reforms often do, by a kind of accident. Among the ill-conducted asylums of this country at that time, the worst seems to have been that of the city of York, which had been founded in 1772, and had soon become a scene of mercenary intrigue and mismanagement. At a much later period it had arrived at the perfection of whatever was wrong and detestable. But, so early as 1791, it happened that a female patient, of the Society of Friends, was placed in this institution. As her family lived at a distance from York, they requested some of their acquaintances to visit her. These acquaintances were denied admission; and in a few weeks the unhappy patient died. This circumstance gave rise to uncomfortable suspicions; or rather it confirmed suspicions which had for some time existed. The Society of Friends, abstaining from any direct reflection on the asylum, acted with their characteristic benevolence and promptness, and, although scarcely able to command sufficiently ample resources, resolved to institute an asylum of their own.

The result was the foundation of the Retreat at York; which was opened a few years afterward. Of this admirable asylum, the first in Europe in which every enlightened principle of treatment was carried into effect, the chief promoter was the late William Tuke of York. His worthy grandson, Samuel Tuke, who is still living, has continued,

C

up to a very advanced period of life, to be a frequent visitor and most active governor of that admirable establishment; and for readers desirous to know the views which ought to prevail in all lunatic asylums, I could not even now refer to any work in which they are more perspicuously explained than in Samuel Tuke's account of the Retreat at York, published in 1813. In the valuable works of Pinel and his honoured successor Esquirol, we find graphic descriptions of all varieties of mental disorders, and lucid views of treatment; but in none are the details of management, economic, medical, and moral, of an institution for the insane, to be found more convincingly set forth than in the work of Samuel Tuke. The substitution of sympathy for gross unkindness, severity, and "stripes;" the diversion of the mind from its excitements and griefs by various occupations; and a wise confidence in the patients when they promised to control themselves, led to the prevalence of order and neatness, and nearly banished furious mania from this wisely devised place of recovery.

All of us who have followed in the path of William and Samuel Tuke, at however great a distance, must ever gratefully acknowledge the extent of our debt to them. It is true that neither they nor Pinel ventured wholly to abolish mechanical coercion; this was left for Charlesworth to attempt, and for Gardiner Hill to carry out, at Lincoln, and for Hanwell to confirm on the largest scale; but when the emulation produced by the changes made in asylums during the last twenty years has subsided, every historian of these establishments must point to Pinel and to Tuke as the men who led the way for the more complete system of non-restraint.

It would be satisfactory to be able to report, that after the exertions of these great and good men, in France and in England, there had been an even course of amelioration in the treatment of lunatics either in one country or the other. Such was not the course in either. Nearly forty years after the reformation began in the asylums of Paris, most of those in the departments continued to present the shocking features formerly characteristic of all. The cells were still narrow, damp, and dark, and some of them underground; air and light being only admitted when the door—four feet or a little more in height—was opened. The furious maniacs slept on the ground, and the helpless lay on straw, seldom renewed; the attendants were still slovenly in appearance, and brutal in manners, and entered the cells armed with sticks, whips, and heavy keys, and accompanied by savage dogs.

Esquirol, who succeeded Pinel at the Salpêtrière in 1810, visited almost every asylum in France; and by his representations of their condition, and by his influence as a physician, and as the first to commence the instruction of students in the management of mental disorders, he effected incalculable benefits throughout France, and it may be said throughout Europe. Writing in 1818, he says, he found the insane naked, or covered with rags, and only protected by straw from the cold damp pavement on which they were lying. They were coarsely fed, without fresh air, without light, without water to allay their thirst, under the dominion of jailors, and chained in caves to which wild beasts would not have been consigned. The general employment of chains was revolting; the patients had collars and belts of iron, and fetters on their hands and feet. Some were fastened to the wall by a chain a foot and a half long, and this method was extolled as being peculiarly calming. Chains were universally preferred to strait-waistcoats, because they were less expensive. There was no medical treatment directed to the cure of the mental malady; and the rude attendants employed seclusion and baths of surprise, and occasional floggings at will.*

The insane were not much better treated in England. Even so late as in the year 1815, such abuses were general.† There is clear proof of their continued existence in 1827; and it cannot be

---

* Des Maladies Mentales, vol. ii., p. 399, 412.

† Report, together with the Minutes of Evidence, &c., from the Committee appointed to consider of Provision being made for the better Regulation of Madhouses in England. London, 1815.

denied that not a few of them survived, in some
public and private asylums, in 1850. The successive
reports of the Commissioners in Lunacy abound in
incontestible and curious evidence of this.   In
some provincial licensed houses the male and female
patients were left at night in miserable outhouses,
without attendants, and without available aid of
any kind; without fire or any means of warmth,
and without protection.   There were no baths;
and no medical treatment was resorted to.   In some
of the largest private asylums near London, the
rooms are described as having been " crowded, wet,
filthy, unventilated, and very offensive," and the
dormitories were lighted and aired by apertures
without glass.   Feeble patients were left without
drink, or any decent attendance; a few potatoes
being given to them now and then, in a wooden
bowl.   In a house at Fonthill, in Wiltshire, out of
14 male patients, only one was without fetters or
handcuffs, and only three were out of their sleeping
rooms.

In another large private asylum, near London,
" several of the pauper women were chained to
their bedsteads, naked, or only covered with
an hempen rug; and this in the month of
December."   From Saturday night till Monday
morning, dirty patients were chained to their cribs,
and confined without intermission " in crowded, ill-
ventilated places."   In these cribs they lay " naked

upon straw, with nothing but a blanket to cover them;" and the window was an aperture without glass. There was no classification, no employment, no medical treatment, no bath, no cleanliness. One towel a week was accorded for the use of 170 patients, and some were mopped with cold water, in the severest weather. As a fitting part of this system, seventy out of about four hundred patients were almost invariably in irons. And this was less than thirty years ago.

Later still, in 1844, the Commissioners reported that in one of the private asylums visited by them, some of the rooms were almost dark; that in some rooms there were neither tables nor seats; that there was not a single change of linen, either for beds or the person, in the whole house. Of course restraints were freely employed, and sometimes the restrained patients had no clothes on. In other private institutions, the violent and the tranquil, the cleanly and the uncleanly, were shut up together: all kinds of mechanical restraints were habitually used, and worn by many who were perfectly quiet. The rooms were dirty, and in some cases insufferably offensive; and airing grounds or gardens there were none.

As recently even as 1846, we find notices in the Commissioners' Reports of the miserable diet allowed in some of the licensed houses. From four and a half ounces of bread to six ounces, with skimmed milk, constituted the breakfast and supper; and what was called a meat and potatoe pie was the dinner; three days in the week, the proportion of meat being less than an ounce for each patient. On two other days the dinner was soup and suet-pudding, and on the remaining two days of the week, when the dinner was called a meat-dinner, the quantity of meat allowed for each patient was only about one ounce and a half. Every thing in the houses corresponded with this parsimony. The passages were extremely cold; the day-rooms had very insufficient fires; one rug and a sheet formed the night-covering of the cribs in which the patients slept; and the day-clothing was often ragged and dirty.

For full seven years, when these things still continued common, the non restraint system had been established at Hanwell. The indifference, or rather the aversion, of the proprietors of these wretched places-to all the means of improving the condition of the unhappy creatures committed to their charge, and their determination to make mechanical restraints a substitute for all better means of control, were, during those years, actively and sometimes triumphantly expressed. The notices of the Commissioners, and the force of public opinion, at length compelled them to reluctant reforms; but the principles which led to all the former abuses have not become extinct, nor can anything but continued vigilance of inspection secure the insane from a recurrence, to a certain extent, to the disgraceful practices of the old mad-houses—for still, of all passions, avarice is the most cruel.

Although the Retreat at York soon acquired a high character, the old York Asylum still continued to be a disgrace to that great county, and to the country at large; its management advancing from one enormity to another, until, in 1813, after years of honourable struggle on the part of a few independent country gentlemen, who were not daunted by the indignant resolutions of the committee, or by continued eulogies of the Asylum from noblemen of the highest influence, the whole system was at length exposed to day.

Secresy had long been the protection of the officers. The physicians administered medicines of which the nature was concealed. Visitors were, as much as possible, excluded. The committee of managers were equally arrogant and ignorant. Every abuse reigned uncontrolled. The poorer patients were half starved. There was no classification within doors or without. Cleanliness and ventilation were disregarded. Numbers of patients were huddled together in small day-rooms. Some slept three in a bed. The use of chains seems to have been very general. The actual *disappearance* of many patients was never accounted for; and some were supposed to have been killed. In reporting the number of deaths, several—sometimes 100 out of 300—were taken from the list of dead, and placed in the list of cured. A general system of dishonesty and peculation prevailed. The physician was dishonest; the steward falsified his accounts and burnt his books; and the matron, a worthy coadjutor, made a profit on the articles purchased by her for the use of the house.

Pending the inquiry into these and various other acts of impropriety and cruelty, an attempt was made, very consistently, and evidently with the knowledge of the officers, to destroy the whole building by fire—books, papers, and patients. To a certain extent the design was successful. Much of the building,was consumed, with most of the books and papers; and several of the patients—it was never ascertained how many—perished at the same time.

It was not until 1814 that the iniquities of this bad place were finally put a stop to. It was not even until that year that secret cells were first discovered by Mr. Godfrey Higgins, one of the most indefatigable of reformers—cells, many in number, and, as his report represented, "in a state of filth horrible beyond description."* The very existence of these cells had been kept from

* A History of the York Asylum, &c. York, 1815. A work ascribed, I believe correctly, to the late Mr. Jonathan Gray.

the knowledge of the committee up to that time.

The following year, 1815, is memorable in the annals of asylums, as that in which the attention of Parliament was directed to the state of Bethlem Hospital. The good seed sown at York had now begun to produce fruit. Samuel Tuke's work was published in 1813; and it was reviewed, in 1814, in the *Edinburgh Review*, by the Rev. Sydney Smith, whose powerful and witty pen was often devoted to objects of the purest philanthropy. In the same year, Mr. Wakefield, Mr. Western, and Mr. Calvert visited Bethlem Hospital, the state of which Mr. Wakefield described to a Committee of the House of Commons in May, 1815. In referring to this Report, it must be remembered that we have now arrived at a period twenty-three years after Pinel's reform.

In the women's galleries in Bethlem they found in one of the side rooms "about ten patients, each chained by one arm or leg to the wall; the chain allowing them merely to stand up by the bench or form fixed to the wall, or to sit down on it." For a dress, each had only a sort of blanket-gown, made like a dressing-gown, but with nothing to fasten it round the body. The feet were without shoes or stockings. Some of these patients were lost in imbecility, dirty, and offensive; associated with them were others capable of coherent conversation, and sensible and accomplished. Many women were locked up in their cells, chained, without clothing, and with only one blanket for a covering. In the men's wing, six patients in the side room were chained close to the wall, five were handcuffed, and one was locked to the wall by the right arm, as well as by the right leg. Except the blanket-gown, these men had no clothing; the room had the appearance of a dog-kennel. Chains were universally substituted for the strait-waistcoat. Those who were not cleanly, and all who were disinclined to get up, were allowed to lie in bed; in what state may be imagined. In one cell they found a patient, a representation of whose condition is preserved in a plate published in Esquirol's work, not much to the honour of our English treatment. This patient's name was Norris. He had been a powerful and violent man. Having on one occasion resented what he considered some improper treatment by his keeper, he was fastened by a long chain, which was ingeniously passed through a wall into the next room, where the victorious keeper, out of the patient's reach, could drag the unfortunate man close to the wall whenever he pleased. To prevent this sort of outrage, poor Norris muffled the chain with straw; but the savage inclinations of the keeper were either checked by no superintending eye, or the officers of the asylum partook of his cruelty and his fears: for now a new and refined torture for the patient was invented, in the shape of an ingenious apparatus of iron. " A stout iron ring was riveted round his neck, from which a short chain passed to a ring made to slide upwards or downwards on an upright massive iron bar, more than six feet high, inserted into the wall. Round his body a strong iron bar, about two inches wide, was riveted: on each side of the bar was a circular projection which, being fastened to, and enclosing each of his arms, pinioned them close to his sides."

The effect of this apparatus was, that the patient could indeed raise himself up so as to stand against the wall, but could not stir one foot from it, could not walk one step, and could not even lie down, except on his back; and in this thraldom he had lived for twelve years. During much of that time he is reported to have been rational in his conversation. But for him, in all those twelve years, there had been no variety of any kind, no refreshing change, no relief: no fresh air; no exercise; no sight of fields or gardens, or earth, or heaven. Each miserable day was like another, and each night. At length release came, which he only lived about a year to enjoy. It is painful to have to add, that this long-continued punishment had the recorded approbation of all the authorities of the hospital. Nothing can more forcibly illustrate the hardening effect of being habitual witnesses of cruelty, and the process which the heart of man undergoes when allowed to exercise irresponsible power. Partly from custom, and partly from indifference, and partly from fear, even physicians not particularly chargeable with inhumanity, used formerly to see patients in every form of irritating restraint, and leave them as they found them. Such facts justify the extremest jealousy of admitting the slightest occasional appliance of mechanical restraints in any asylum. Once admitted, under whatever pretext, and every abuse will follow in time.

To turn from these horrors, and to record improvement and advance, and the triumph of kindness and judgment over severity and brute force, is a relief to the mind. But it is well to remember that almost every enormity continued to prevail, so long as mechanical restraints continued to be habitually employed in asylums, and that the abolition of these lingering abuses only steadily proceeded when mechanical restraints were abandoned. From 1792 to 1839 every variety of neglect continued to be observed and reported as existing in most of the public and private asylums ; from the latter date, when mechanical coercion was first totally abolished in a few of our large asylums, all such abuses have been gradually disappearing ; and the non-restraint system having in the course of fifteen years become the rule, the abuses, like mechanical restraints, have become the exception.

It is now sixteen years since the use of all mechanical restraints was abolished, first at Lincoln, then at Hanwell—a change which, soon after adopted at Northampton, Glasgow, Lancaster, Gloucester, and Stafford, led by degrees to the establishment of a system of treatment comprehending a great variety of particulars, successively and considerately devised as substitutes for bonds and fetters and all kinds of mechanical coercion. This system, opposed to the practice of centuries, to many prejudices, and to many purely selfish feelings, has since that period steadily, although slowly, advanced, until from almost every public asylum in England, Scotland, and Ireland, mechanical restraints have been wholly excluded. Wherever the attempt has been resolutely made it has succeeded; and of the many new and splendid lunatic asylums built and opened in England within the last eight years there does not appear to be one into which any instrument of mechanical restraint has yet found admission.

It is, still, in our country only that this amelioration has found perfect favour. Over a great part of the continent of Europe it has been warmly opposed, and is still opposed, although not tried. It has been elaborately discussed and especially condemned in important official reports in France; and some recent reports of one or two of our English asylums have contained expressions indicative of a willingness to recur to the use of restraints, on pretences so slight as to show that the gradual reappearance of all the dreadful apparatus of mechanical coercion is within the limits of possibility.

Of course even the strongest advocates of mechanical restraint in this country are sufficiently prudent not to outrage the feelings of visitors by any striking exhibition of it. If it exists in some melancholy apartments in their houses, these apartments are not generally exhibited; and all that is professed is a moderate recourse to methods maintained to be sometimes indispensable. But no fallacy can be greater than that of imagining what is called a moderate use of mechanical restraint to be consistent with a general plan of treatment in all other respects complete, and unobjectionable, and humane. The abolition must be absolute, or it cannot be efficient. Possible cases of exception may occur, although scarcely in public asylums. But, generally, if hands and feet are allowed, as the ordinary practice and custom of the asylum, to be tied and bound at the will of the attendants, all forms of deterioration will appear in the patients, and all kinds of neglect and tyranny will be engendered; until, by slow but very sure steps, restraints become the usual substitutes for attention, for patience, for forbearance, and proper superintendence.

The very recent exposure, by the Commissioners

in Lunacy, of the manner in which the insane paupers are treated in the workhouses of London, has produced facts which fully prove that all the old evils are only kept in check by superintendence and publicity; and that the tendency to neglect those who are deprived of reason still exists, and demands vigilant opposition. What the old system of treatment by restraint really was ought, therefore, not to be forgotten, nor should palliations of it be unreflectingly admitted. Its evils were not imaginary, but real and dreadful. In the clean, quiet, orderly galleries of well managed asylums, the visitor now sees nothing indicative of the condition to which the apologists of restraints look back as scarcely objectionable. In the gloomy mansions in which hands and feet were daily bound with straps or chains, and wherein chairs of restraint, and baths of surprise, and even whirling-chairs were tolerated, all was consistently bad. The patients were a defenceless flock, at the mercy of men and women who were habitually severe, often cruel, and sometimes brutal. The evidence of this stands on record, and can neither be denied or explained away. Cold apartments, beds of straw, meagre diet, scanty clothing, scanty bedding, darkness, pestilent air, sickness and suffering, and medical neglect — all these were common ; and they must remain common, however disguised, wherever the system of restraint remains the subject of eulogy. Before the appointment of commissioners, armed with power to inspect these receptacles of madness, there was so much security and concealment that the aggravations of loathsome dirt, of swarming vermin, and of the keeper's lash, were safely added. No mercy, no pity, no decent regard for affliction, for age, or for sex, existed. Old and young, men and women, the frantic and the melancholy, were treated worse, and more neglected, than the beasts of the field. The cells of an asylum resembled the dens of a squalid menagerie : the straw was raked out, and the food was thrown in through the bars ; and exhibitions of madness were witnessed which are no longer to be found, because they were not the simple product of malady, but of malady aggravated by mismanagement. I refrain from an unnecessary accumulation of details in proof of assertions, some of which, in these better days, may appear exaggerated; but several are to be found in the Parliamentary Report of 1815, and in the various Reports of the Commissioners already cited; and in a small work published in Edinburgh, in 1837, by Dr. W. A. F. Browne, the physician to the Crichton Royal Institution for Lunatics at Dumfries, entitled " What asylums were, are, and ought to be ; " and also in a volume published in London in 1850, by the late medical superintendent of an asylum for the insane, called

"Familiar Views of Lunacy and Lunatic Life."
The article "Lunatic Asylums" in the "Supplement
to the Penny Cyclopædia" contains other facts
and references in relation to the same subjects.

PART II.

THE FIRST DAYS OF THE NEW OR NON-RESTRAINT SYSTEM.

As the restraint system comprehended every possible evil of bad treatment, every fault of commission and omission, so the watchful, preventive, almost parental superintendence included in the term non-restraint, creates guards against them all. For such is its real character, if properly understood and practised. It is, indeed, above all, important to remember, and it is the principal object of this work to explain, that the mere abolition of fetters and restraints constitutes only a part of what is properly called the non-restraint system. Accepted in its full and true sense, it is a complete system of management of insane patients, of which the operation begins the moment a patient is admitted over the threshold of an asylum. To describe the whole system successfully, we must imagine the case of a maniacal patient just brought to the reception-room. We must suppose this to be in an asylum wherein a good system has already been established, and that the attendants are efficient and respectable, and the whole establishment is well arranged; that the diet is liberal, the clothing is clean, and the general aspect of the place cheerful. These are conditions seldom or never found in asylums where mechanical restraints are retained. The attendants in such places have a peculiar character: the female attendants are generally morose in aspect, and slatterns; and the male attendants, ill-dressed and ill-mannered, have the appearance of ruffians. The clothing of the patients is scanty and ragged; the food is ill prepared and coarse; the rooms are often offensive to sight and smell; and discomfort and gloom prevail everywhere.

But I must be permitted to suppose a case admitted at Hanwell; a place which I know the best, and can speak of the most positively. The case may be that of a man who for a week or two has been violently maniacal; who, becoming first, perhaps, idle and intemperate, has terrified his family, broken the furniture of his house, or attacked his neighbours; or harangued the public and disturbed the streets, and resisted all control until overcome by the police. He comes to the asylum bound very tightly, sometimes hand and foot, or fastened in a strait-waistcoat. He is still violent, but exhausted; he is flushed, feverish, thirsty; in appearance haggard, and in manner fierce, or sullen. His voice is hoarse with shouting. He is unwashed, unshaved, and half starved. His clothes are torn and dirty. He has often many bruises or injuries, which he has incurred in his furious condition. His violence is still dreaded, and he exhibits capricious proofs of remaining strength; so that those who have brought him to the asylum are afraid to stay, and unfeignedly rejoice to get rid of him; wondering that any people should be found to take charge of him, and earnestly warning them to take care of themselves.

Or the case may be that of a female patient, equally violent, but whose frantic exertions proceed from a dread she entertains that some fearful punishment is impending over her; that she is to be cut to pieces, or to be burned alive; and this for crimes of which she believes herself to be accused. With these impressions, her thoughts are probably bent on suicide, as an expiation, or as a means of escape from sufferings. Cases of infinite variety may be imagined; in all of which confusion, and bewilderment, and terror under all surrounding circumstances, for a time disturb the mind. In all these cases, the first difficulties appear so great, and the dangers so pressing, that the idea of mere security naturally predominates in the bystanders;

and this would seem to be most readily obtained
by continuing the restraints, and superadding
seclusion and darkness. These ready means were
formerly wholly relied upon ; and starvation, dirt,
and severities of many kinds as naturally followed
in their train. But it is a part of the non-restraint
system to remember, whatever the state and
circumstances of a newly admitted patient may
be, that he comes to the asylum to be cured, or, if
incurable, to be protected and taken care of, and
kept out of mischief, and tranquillized ; and that
the strait-waistcoat effects none of these objects.
Therefore, although the patients may arrive bound
so securely as scarcely to be able to move, they are
at once released from every ligature and bond and
fetter that may have been imposed upon them.
They appear generally to be themselves surprised at
this proceeding ; and for a time are tranquil, yet
often distrustful, and uncertain in their movements.
Now and then the tranquillising effect of this
unexpected liberty is permanent: more frequently
it is but temporary. But every newly admitted
patient is as soon as possible visited by the medical
officers of the asylum. They assure the stranger,
by a few kind words, that no ill-treatment is any
longer to be feared. This assurance sometimes gains
the confidence of the patient at once, and is ever
afterward remembered: but in many cases the patient
is too much confused to be able to comprehend it.

Few or none, however, are quite insensible to the measures immediately adopted in conformity to it.

The wretched clothes are removed; the patient is taken gently to the bath-room, and has, probably for the first time, the comfort of a warm-bath; which often occasions expressions of remarkable satisfaction. The refreshed patient is taken out of the bath, carefully dried, and has clean and comfortable clothing put on : he is then led to the day-room, and offered good and well prepared food. The very plates, and knife and fork, and all the simple furniture of the table, are cleaner by far than what he has lately been accustomed to, or perhaps such as in his miserable struggling life he never knew before. A patient seen after these preliminary parts of treatment is scarcely to be recognised as the same patient who was admitted only an hour before. The non-restraint treatment has commenced; and some of its effects already appear.

But the patient may be too much absorbed in delusions, or too much occupied by anger, or by fear alone, to derive immediate benefit even from these parts of a kind reception, or to admit of being consoled by the kindest words, or, for a time, carefully medically examined. This state will not last very long, if no severity and no neglect are permitted. Whilst it does last, the efforts of the officers are limited to such measures as ensure the

safety of the patient and of those surrounding
him, and which also contribute to the return of
calmness.   The patients, however, are often merely
restless and fidgetty ; run about ; or are inclined to
acts of harmless mischief: and in such cases much
interference merely irritates them.   One of the
things which attendants are slowest to learn is not
to interfere unnecessarily. If every movement of
the patient is checked, and every impulse thwarted,
the patient, good tempered before, becomes angry,
and   strikes   the   attendant : and   such,   where
restraints are employed, is the frequent cause of
the first imposition of a strait-waistcoat.   I have
known many patients brought to the asylum whose
first days there were passed in violence which
would have been protracted by their being fastened
by leather and iron, and yet who could not be at
large during those few days without dangers being
incurred.   Two very erroneous representations of
our method of management in such cases have been
repeated very often ; and have neither yielded to
the most positive contradiction, nor to what the
visitors to asylums might have learnt from their
own observation.

One is, that although we abstain from the use of
any form of mechanical restraint, we substitute for
such restraints the muscular force of strong-armed
attendants, who hold fast the refractory patients for
a long time together.   The impossibility of such

a proceeding would seem self-evident; but the advocates of the old restraints have perpetually availed themselves of the argument; very reasonably observing that such a practice would be as actual a form of restraint as a strait waistcoat, but very unreasonably failing to observe that no such practice is resorted to. In every foreign publication, intended to defend the continued employment of the camisole, this argument is repeated, year after year, even by those writers who have visited English asylums, and who insist on the prevalence of a practice which they never could have witnessed. The truth is, that repression by holding the patients' hands and arms is never resorted to except when some sudden impulse requires such immediate interposition for a few minutes, after which the impulse usually passes away; or the patient is removed, and his attention occupied with something that makes him forget it. Against such sudden impulses it would never be right to resort to mechanical restraint; and any continued holding, or struggling, or violent overmastering of an irritable patient belongs to the older system of treatment, and is quite inconsistent with the new.

The other representation is that, although we do not fasten hand or foot, we place our violent patients in solitary confinement. This unfortunate expression originated with the Commissioners in

Lunacy, in one of their Reports many years ago. The Commissioners, since that time, have so steadily discountenanced the use of mechanical restraints, that I should not advert to this mistaken description of what is really resorted to, if short occasional seclusion was not a medicine, and if the padded rooms, the real substitutes for restraints in very violent cases, were not of the highest importance—offering, indeed, an auxiliary, without which it is questionable whether or not restraints could be entirely dispensed with in any large asylum.

In the Reports presented within the last few years to the Prefect of the Département de la Seine, already referred to, restraints are very ingeniously defended, but altogether on erroneous premises. In the second, it is assumed that the padded rooms are used in England to meet every difficulty; and that the French system, which applies the camisole to meet slight evils, and the seclusion-room to meet graver, is better than ours, which comprehends the sole resource of seclusion. But it is overlooked that with us seclusion is only employed when the patient cannot be at large with benefit to himself, or with safety to others; and that all other difficulties are met without using the camisole—met by watching and care, and well devised clothing, and various resources, none of which irritate the patient, or render him helpless or uncleanly, as the strait-waistcoat always must do. It is also to be remembered that the French seclusion-rooms are not padded, or at all fitted up like ours.

Many English superintendents speak of seclusion as something worse than mechanical restraint; seeming to forget that it is as much adapted to secure an irritable brain from causes of increased irritability as a quiet chamber and the exclusion of glare, and of many visitors, is adapted to the same state of brain in a fever. The patient needs repose, and every object, or every person seen, irritates him. No physician of experience in cases of insanity can be unacquainted with the tendency to exhaustion and death in all recent cases of violent insanity—a tendency which struggling with restraints, or the continued excitements unavoidable in a crowd of lunatics, greatly increases, and which silence and rest can alone obviate. It is often seen that the mere moving of the cover of the inspection-plate in the door of a patient's room, if not cautiously done, rouses the patient from tranquillity, and causes him to start up and rush violently to the door. When let alone he lies down again. Seclusion gives him the benefit of continued tranquillity, by removing at once every cause of excitement. He sits in his own bed-room instead of sitting exposed to a crowd of patients. The superintendents who condemn seclusion as if it were a mere punishment would find, I believe, if they passed more hours in their wards, that by many an afflicted patient, silence and retirement are the blessings most anxiously desired.

Sometimes the same absence of excitement is obtained by allowing patients to walk about alone in one of the airing courts, and this is always resorted to as soon as it is practicable. The form of delusion under which the patient labours may make this impossible. He may mistake those whom he sees for those who are absent, and who are the objects of his suspicion or dislike ; or he may think that the devil is approaching him, in the shape of one of the patients near him. Violent attacks, serious accidents, and even homicides, have been the consequence of such delusions, in many asylums; and the best security against such accidents is quietness, or the temporary isolation of excited patients, or, in other words, seclusion in a padded room, which includes both advantages.

The great advantage of a padded room in all these cases, is that it renders both mechanical restraints and muscular force unnecessary for the control of even the most violent patients. Such an apartment, at Hanwell, is prepared by a thick soft padding of coir (cocoa-nut fibre), enclosed in ticken, fastened to wooden frames, and affixed to the four walls of the room—the padding extending from the floor to a height above the ordinary reach of a patient. The whole floor of the room is padded also, or covered with a thick mattress, of the same material as the padded walls, so that it makes a complete bed.   In general, the room contains no furniture except bolsters or pillows, also covered with strong ticken.   The window is guarded by a close wire-blind, which admits light and air, but prevents access on the part of the patient to the glass or window frames.   If the patient is disposed to suicide, the clothing he wears is of a strength and consistence resisting his efforts to tear it into strings to effect his purpose, and the blankets are enclosed in strong ticken cases.   In a room so arranged the patient cannot easily injure himself, or receive accidental injury.   Nor is he left to chance. The seclusion, and the reasons for it, are always immediately reported to the superintendent or physician, and, in the case of female patients, to the matron also.   The ward is visited from time to time by these officers, and an accurate knowledge of the state of the secluded patient is obtained by means of an inspection-plate or covered opening in the door of the room.   The patient is not left to suffer from thirst or hunger, nor are his personal state and cleanliness unattended to; nor is he allowed to remain in seclusion longer than his excited state requires.   A written report of each instance of seclusion, and of its duration, is sent to the physician at the close of each day, and copied by him into a book which is inspected at every meeting of the Committee.   Thus are obtained all the advantages of seclusion, without any abuse of it.

Seclusion is also effected without violence, which the imposition of a strait-waistcoat can seldom be. If the newly arrived patient is perfectly unreasonable and unmanageable whilst at large, he is not left to be overpowered by one or even by two attendants. A number of attendants are quietly assembled ; they attract the patient's attention, and often succeed in persuading him to go into his own bedroom, or into a padded apartment, of his own accord. If he resists the most patient persuasion, or defies the attendants altogether, they are trained to effect the seclusion without a contest, or even more than a momentary struggle. After all words have failed, they close quickly upon him, and three or four of them catch hold of him at once, and so dexterously that he can scarcely either kick or strike them; and he is carried into the room like a child, and dropped gently on his bed or on the padded floor. The attendants make a hasty retreat, lock the door, and leave the patient in a solitude which seems to surprise him. Usually, he soon becomes calm, and gradually he becomes good humoured and approachable. Very generally, he lies quiet for a time, and then falls asleep. If he continues violent, he can neither hurt himself nor anybody else. If he remains turbulent and noisy, he disturbs nobody. In time

he always becomes more tranquil, and any approach
to tranquillity is watched for, as the opportunity of
offering him food, or cold water to drink, or tea, or
broth, or refreshment of various kinds, and of attending to all his requirements, and conciliating him.   A
good-tempered attendant now succeeds in making
acquaintance with him; and as soon as the least
reason returns to the patient, he begins to understand that he has got to some place where the
people are kind to him.   He sees that he is visited
with good intentions only, and having no rankling
recollection of ill-treatment of any sort, he grows
friendly with the attendants, becomes docile, and
thanks them.   The cure has commenced.

This method of meeting the various difficulties
to be overcome in maniacal cases is plainly enough
preferable to the methods formerly employed, and
under which, a refractory patient would have
been forcibly invested with an uncomfortable and
irritating strait-waistcoat, and then, perhaps, shut
up in a dark room, not padded, and having no
resting-place but an iron crib without bedding,
in which he would also probably have been fastened
down.   Every possible evil of seclusion was then
combined with every suffering incidental to the
confinement of the arms and the legs, and the whole
body; and the patient, excited and feverish from
his malady, and heated and exasperated by the
previous struggle, was left to lie in a constrained

and comfortless position, and to suffer thirst, and
to become subjected to all the miseries of unavoidable uncleanliness. With such treatment the
patient commonly became furious. All kind
attentions being incompatible with such disregard
and neglect of him, there was no avenue to a good
understanding between him and the attendants,
whom he then, and long afterward, only looked
upon as his enemies and tormentors. The superintendents who speak of padded rooms as useless,
do not explain their present mode of treating
very violent patients in the recent stages of mania.
What it used to be when no padded rooms were
employed is well known to me, and there are
patients now living who can too well remember
it. At that time, when a young and accomplished
woman for example, affected with acute mania,
violent, noisy, mischievous, regardless of cleanliness,
arrived at a large asylum, she was forcibly undressed,
fastened down on loose straw, had strong medicine
forced down her throat, and was then left and
neglected for many hours. The straw tortured
her from head to foot, but she could not move
her hands. Her position galled and fretted her;
but her feet were fastened, and she could not
change it. Sickness and purging were produced
by the medicine; and she was permitted to lie
for twelve hours in a state of indescribable distress,
then taken up, laid on the stone pavement, mopped

or broomed, and last of all, when quite subdued and half dead, had, perhaps, a bath, and some few decent attentions.

Such an example occurs to my recollection as having been afterward recorded by the patient herself. Where there are no padded rooms to resort to, I fear some parts of this ancient treatment must be scarcely avoidable; for many patients, particularly in the early stage of their malady, cannot safely be at large in the wards except in close restraints, nor safely placed in an ordinary sleeping-room, unless they are fastened to the bedstead. This state may continue for many days, or sometimes for many weeks; and for meeting such exigencies, the padded room, and much watching, and all practicable attentions seem alone adapted.

The effects produced by a good or bad reception, and the influence of impressions made during the first few days passed in an asylum, on the various cases received—the violent, the despairing, the timid, the imbecile—may be easily imagined. Sometimes, indeed, all the worst features of the cases disappear so speedily as to make their previously recorded character scarcely credible. A man reported dirty and violent has sometimes himself remarked, when accidentally seeing these characters written on his admission-paper, that he might well be both when he was fastened down in a trough, half fed, and often struck; and

E

such patients, on being set at liberty, have not unfrequently at once become cleanly in their habits and calm in their conduct. Even in asylums for patients far above the rank of paupers, the kindness, and cleanliness, and general comfort of a good asylum are strongly appreciated. I have repeatedly known private patients, received from some of the worst of the old-fashioned establishments, reported to be incurably dirty, or violent, or dangerous; the true explanation being that such patients had been kept much in bed, and often in darkness, having neither a due supply of good food, nor a proper change of dress: for the richest patients, and those of highest rank, may, no less than the poor, be subjected to such indignities and shameful neglect. In these circumstances they become fretful, negligent of cleanliness, reckless, and often violent. Amidst the wildness of madness, they are still, to a certain extent, sensible of their degraded position; and every feeling is concentrated into hatred of everybody about them or connected with them. An officer of rank in a distinguished cavalry regiment, came to an asylum with which I am acquainted, from one in which a more than commonly obstinate attachment had been maintained in favour of restraints, and maintained for many years. His whole wardrobe consisted of two shirts, one nightshirt, two pairs of stockings, one pair of drawers, and the clothes which he daily wore, and which were old, dirty, and ragged. He appeared to be surprised when shown into a well-furnished room, and quite astonished when he saw a comfortable dinner before him, and when his tea was decently served in the evening. Patients who have been so negligently cared for, almost always improve when thus respectfully and kindly treated. They make an effort to conform to the decent habits of the house; are more careful to be cleanly when their dress is no longer the dress of a beggar; and become civil and even courteous in their demeanour. The violent conduct which caused them to be fastened in restraints in the old establishment disappears amongst the comforts of their new and better abode; and thus, with the abolition of preliminary negligences, mechanical restraint is found to be unnecessary, and all its attendant evils are abolished also.

In the greater number of recent cases of mental malady the patient is unable to sleep; the days are tolerably tranquil, but with the night restless distraction comes. Whoever has known the affliction of a restless night must know that his affliction would have received no abatement from his being tied down to his bed; and that fresh air, cold water, sitting up awhile, and diversion of mind, are the things to which he would resort for relief. The poor lunatic, equally restless, equally sleepless, and with a brain more excited, should not be deprived of these alleviations, all of which form a part of the true non-restraint system; but none of which are regarded where restraints are employed, which are, indeed, utterly incompatible with them. The attendant who has fastened down his troublesome and sleepless patients in bed, retires, with a satisfied mind, to his supper and his rest. The patients may suffer from heat and thirst, and may shout and yell in their despair— he heeds them not; or, if he does, it is only to visit them in an angry mood, and to punish them as he chooses. The attendant, where restraints are not used, cannot leave his patients so neglected, or punish them at will. The physician himself, in large asylums, frequently goes round the wards at night, and a system is established by which their state is reported to him every morning. If a patient cannot lie down without distress, he is not compelled to lie down, but allowed to walk about; being supplied with soft warm shoes and other clothing, to prevent his suffering from being out of bed. If he knocks at the door of his room, the reason of his doing so is inquired into; if he is thirsty, he has water given to him; if he has been restless, and his bed is discomposed, the bed is made comfortable again; the patient's face and hands are cooled with water; perhaps a cup of tea, or coffee, or beef-tea, or arrow-root—kept

in readiness by the night attendants—is given
to him, or sometimes a little tobacco; and thus
the patient is refreshed in body and soothed in
mind, blesses his visitors, bids them good-night,
and falls asleep; and thus, the cries and howls
which disturbed the wards so often are heard no
more.

The old system placed all violent or troublesome patients in the position of dangerous animals·
The new system regards them as afflicted persons,
whose brain and nerves are diseased, and who are
to be restored to health, and comfort, and reason.
This simple difference of view it is which influences
every particular in the arrangement of every part
of an asylum for the insane.

Thus, whilst in the old asylums every arrangement
was principally made for security and control, in
the new, every arrangement is made for the cure of
the malady, or the comfort of the insane.   In many
of the old asylums there were even no infirmaries.
Many patients, admitted in states of suffering and
danger, needing repose, and requiring the utmost
medical care, were placed in or near wards
containing noisy patients; and the medical
arrangements were negligent and slovenly to an
extent which, if described, would scarcely now be
believed.   Ill educated superintendents seemed
afraid to have well-informed medical officers about
them; and such appointments, instead of being, as

they now are, objects of competition among highly accomplished medical men, were usually filled by such as were merely unfit to engage in private practice; ill educated men, of illiberal views, and opposed to every improvement. The mischievous activity of the patients then occupied the whole attention of the officers and keepers; but the distempered brain was forgotten. The institution had closetsful of straps and manacles, but all the accessaries of moral and even of medical treatment were deficient.

Keeping in recollection the newly admitted, it may be readily understood how important it is that all the arrangements of an asylum, both by day and night, should be calculated to calm the troubled spirits of insane persons; that everything should be done regularly, and everything done quietly. Nothing, however, can ensure this but the most systematic supervision of the physician, with the daily aid of efficient and well-disposed male and female officers, exercised over good-tempered, active, well-chosen attendants. Perfect order, perfect cleanliness, and great tranquillity, should prevail everywhere. No excuse should be admitted for a disorderly ward, or a neglected gallery, or for a permanent bad odour in any room in the whole building. In the attempt to establish this condition in an old asylum, every form of ingenious opposition must at first be expected. It will be represented

that some patients are unmanageable; and that
some of the apartments cannot possibly be kept
free from bad odours. These representations are
never to be accepted as excuses. The attendants
must be incited to fresh exertions, and moved to
emulate what is done by others ; and difficulties
which appeared formidable will be found absolutely
to disappear. This cannot be effected unless the
physician himself condescends to details. To
walk through the house, and hear that there is
nothing particular to be reported to him, would be
a useless ceremony. Having in his mind a comprehensive system of treatment, nothing which
forms a part of it is beneath his attention. These
minute particulars are worthy of regard because
they are really therapeutical. We seek a mild air
for the consumptive, and place the asthmatic in an
atmosphere which does not irritate him, and keep
a patient with heart disease on level ground ; and
on the same prophylactic and curative principles,
we must study to remove from an insane person
every influence that can further excite his brain,
and to surround him with such as, acting soothingly
on both body and mind, may favour the brain's
rest, and promote the recovery of its normal
action.

On awaking, in the morning after arrival, in a
strange place, and wholly among strangers, all that
meets the eye and ear of the new patient should be

consolatory, or at least encouraging. To be washed and dressed carefully and patiently, or hastily and roughly—to sit down to a comfortable breakfast, or to have food rudely thrown down on the table—makes all the difference in the patient's feelings that can be imagined. The care observed as to these particulars in a good asylum, and the general quietness and order of the wards, so remarkably influence the newly admitted patients, that for a time, in very many cases, their malady seems almost to have disappeared. This is, of course, most observable in tranquil patients, labouring under delusions ; but it is often manifest in very perturbed cases, and, to a certain extent, in the most depressed, or in the terrified, whose griefs or fears are at once somewhat allayed. The daily visits of the physician and his assistants on the male and female side of the asylum, if those officers are attentive to a duty which is really the most important duty of each day, are even expected with pleasure by all the patients, who feel that they are under protection. These visits should not be formal and hurried ; but time should be given to each ward, and even to many individual patients, whose character for the day will often depend much on these interviews. It is, therefore, important that the officers should dismiss all their own cares from the mind on commencing the morning inspection ; and be ready to hear with patience,

to investigate with justice, and to remedy with
kindness, all the little or great causes of dissatis-
faction laid before them ; so that the patients
may be tranquillised, and, at the same time, the
attendants not ruffled and discomposed, and left in
an unfit state themselves to show kindness or
exercise patience towards others through the rest
of the hours of the day.

To not a few of the newly arrived patients in a
county asylum, the mere circumstance of being
taken into the chapel to prayers is a novelty that
makes a favourable impression on the mind. The
tranquil worship, and the order and neatness which
surround them, are so contrasted with the noisy,
struggling, wrangling, prayerless life they led so
lately, that scarcely any patient is dull enough to be
quite insensible to the change. When, later in the
day, they see the chaplain come into the wards, and
he converses with them gently and judiciously, their
feelings are often evidently touched by a sympathy
to which, even from early childhood, they have
been strangers. When they are taken out to walk
in a quiet garden, or a pleasant field, among trees,
and shrubs, and flowers, they are impressed with
the sensations of a kind of new world. When,
sitting down to comfortable dinners, they find that
some of the officers still come to see that all is
conducted properly, a conviction that they are

carefully looked after necessarily arises in their
thoughts. The afternoon brings its changes or its
rest. The days soon become occupied, by the men
in the various workshops, or in the gardens, or on
the farm; and by the women in the work-rooms, or
the laundry, or the bakehouse, or the busy and
cheerful, and scrupulously clean kitchen. Wherever
they go they meet kind people, and hear kind
words; they are never passed without some recog-
nition, and the face of every officer is the face of
a friend. In the evening, the domestic meal of tea
refreshes them. Their supper and their bed are
not negligently prepared. Day after day these
influences operate, and day by day mental irritation
subsides, and suspicions die, and gloomy thoughts
gradually disperse, and confidence grows and
strengthens, and natural affections re-awake, and
reason returns.

In short, in an asylum conducted on just
principles, and where not only mechanical restraints,
but all kinds of neglect and severity are abolished,
patients of every rank appreciate and benefit by
the change. Those who have been well educated
express themselves in warm terms of satisfaction,
and the poorer classes often convey their simple
gratitude in the most affecting terms. They refer
to their former treatment with horror, and recall,
again and again, the first kind words which they

say they had heard for many years, and which some sympathizing officer or attendant uttered soon after their arrival.

A newly received patient, being brought to a condition of comparative comfort by the mode of reception described, is now capable of deriving benefit from the conversation of the medical superintendent, and generally, from the cheerful aspect of a well governed asylum. Hope, which had abandoned him, begins to return. He sees no wretched patients hobbling about in leg-locks, or, although dressed in strait-waistcoats, which confine their arms, running a-muck at all they meet. He sees no blows inflicted, and hears no taunting and unkind words. The fearful images which lately possessed his mind, of a prison, of punishment, or a cruel death, gradually depart; and sometimes, even at this early period, his recovery seems to commence. Harsh treatment would have confirmed his apprehensions, and have prolonged his violence; so as to have made a resort to mechanical restraints appear excusable. But in a well regulated asylum such modes of restraint are never thought excusable. Each case is studied as soon as the interval of calmness ensues; and means are provided which cause every return of excitement, and every accident or change of the malady, to be met without serious difficulty, and without danger. All this, however, supposes a complete establishment, humane attendants, faithful officers, and a chief physician resolved to allow no excuse for cruelty, or for the indolence which so often leads to cruelty. It demands the constant supervision of efficient officers over attendants, whose duty is positively to obey the physician. If the attendants are not sufficiently numerous, or if the officers have not sufficient authority, or if the discipline required to be daily and hourly observed is relaxed, or can possibly be relaxed by a capricious board or committee, vain of their own power, and not unwilling to humiliate their own officers, the non-restraint system, in pureness and integrity, cannot be maintained. There can be no security for its continuance. The asylum may now and then be dressed up as a place of show; but the condition of the patients, day by day, night by night, hour by hour, may still be rendered unhappy, and many concealed severities practised upon them.

If we were to watch the admissions at the gate of an asylum, we should more fully appreciate the manner in which the system pursued in the establishment applies to them. Not only to the maniacal patient, who comes tied up because he is violent, nor to the melancholic creature who is also tied and bound, because he desires to end his existence, does the non-restraint system bring deliverance and comfort. Many an unhappy patient is brought who is already partially affected with paralysis. In an asylum where mechanical restraints are employed, these patients are first put into restraints because they are mischievous; and after a time they are fastened in a heavy coercion-chair, pierced like a close-stool, because they are helpless and dirty. In some of the old asylums I have seen rows of chairs filled with these poor creatures, in rooms having a sloping floor and gutter, but rooms less clean and comfortable than the generality of stables. They sat in those chairs all the day, and they were fastened down on straw at night. They were rudely washed in the morning—perhaps with a mop; they were carelessly fed; they were clothed in the refuse clothing of the house. It was painfully offensive to approach them, and some of them had even become frantic from neglect and constraint, kicked the boards which enclosed them with impotent violence, yelling out their despair, and were now and then quieted by blows. Sometimes they seized a heedless passer-by, and exercised upon him all their remaining desperate strength. Then they were pronounced dangerous, restraints were accumulated upon them, and their hands were fastened to their sides, or secured with manacles. Perhaps they never breathed the fresh air any more, and their comfort in summer and in winter was no more cared for. Hands and feet blue and icy cold attested their debility and the neglect of it, and mortification of the toes was not a rare result. Growing rapidly weaker, the attendants ceased to take the trouble of getting them out of bed at all, and all their time was passed in a wretched crib, generally wet—their hands and feet being still often fastened. Ulceration of the back frequently ensued, and death alone relieved them from that condition of neglect and woe. I write as if these things were past—in some parts of the Continent they may still be witnessed.

The reception and treatment of a paralytic patient in an asylum where no mechanical restraint is ever resorted to are now far different. Received with kindness, and his limbs at once set at liberty, he may continue mischievous, but he is seldom violent or dangerous. It is sometimes found that ulcerations have already commenced; but as the patient no longer sleeps in dirty straw, nor sits in a coercion-chair, nor is neglected as regards his food and clothing, and as he passes much of his time in the open air, and has wine or porter, or whatever his state requires, the ulcerations are soon checked and healed, the patient's general health improves, he grows stout, and his good humour is scarcely ever interrupted. He lives, indeed, a life of almost entire satisfaction, screened by his very malady from worldly care, and by his position from every privation. For a time the mind is found not to have lost its power of being better exercised;

uncleanly habits are overcome, and violent emotions are controlled. The physician knows that the continuance of these and other symptoms of amendment is not to be relied upon ; and that the progress to the utmost helplessness, and from that to death, although it may be delayed, is inevitable. But in each stage of this sure decline, means of alleviation are thought of. When the patient's step becomes more feeble, he walks with the support of an attendant's arm, or not unfrequently with that of the arm of some fellow patient, steadier than himself. In fine weather he sits out of doors nearly all the day, in a large easy chair, so constructed that no straps or belts are required to prevent his falling out of it. If the weather is cold, his chair is placed near a comfortable fire. The state of his extremities and of his back is daily examined. His food is carefully attended to, and divided for him, and when he can no longer feed himself he is fed like a child. A softer bed becomes necessary to him, and, in a still more advanced stage, a water-bed, on which the last months of his life are passed in a painless childish state, all his faltering expressions breathing gratitude and content.

But patients are not unfrequently brought to asylums so enfeebled by disease and by want of sufficient food, or so disabled by long continued confinement of their limbs, as to be unable to walk. They require to be lifted out of the carriage or cart in which they arrive, and to be carried into the wards and placed on a bed. The life or death of these poor creatures depends on their treatment. According to the old system, a bed of straw, and a strap round the body to prevent the patient falling out of bed, were considered nearly all that was required. Perhaps some broth, or tea, or wine, might be given; but too often it was neglected, and the patient's case was abandoned as hopeless. The various alleviations and comforts essential to a sick and suffering creature were almost all wanting, and the patient died. It is only in asylums where every case is regarded as being admitted for treatment, and, if possible, for cure, that such afflicted persons are carefully and tenderly nursed, washed with tepid water, dressed in decent night-clothes, laid on a comfortable bed, supplied with nourishment at proper intervals during the day, and also, when visited, several times in the night. In many and many a case I have seen attentions like these rewarded by great amendment in the patient's state, and in some by recovery: by the gradual restoration of physical strength, and the gradual return of reason.

Among the improvements yet to be made in the practical department of public asylums, arrangements for what may be called an *individualised* treatment are particularly required. None but those daily familiar with the events of asylums can duly appreciate the great effects of such treatment in special cases. After the first improvement in patients received into the best asylums, some will remain stationary for a length of time without the special attention of an intelligent and watchful attendant, whose duties are almost exclusively confined to such cases. For want of such especial care, the signs of improvement may fade away, and the chance of recovery be lost. Patients who have remained listless and unimproving for months, and who have seemed falling into a state of apathy or imbecility, or even verging on the hopeless state of dementia, in a ward in which they received little personal notice or attention, are seen, in some encouraging instances, when happily transferred to attendants who have more disposition to attend to them, or better opportunities of so doing, or greater aptitude for the task, to awaken from their torpor, to become animated, active, and even industrious. The countenance reassumes intelligent and cheerful expression; a disposition to converse returns; all the mental faculties appear gradually to re-acquire capability of exercise; and, in some cases, entire amendment follows.

It may seem difficult to apply the lesson thus learned to many of the inmates of large asylums;

F

but it may be done, and I have known it done to a considerable proportion of recent cases, and occasionally to those of older date, with results so striking, that I should consider it one of the most desirable advantages to a superintending physician, to have at least one or two superior attendants on each side of the asylum devoted to this duty; the particular cases for its performance being assigned to them by the physician, or by the officers cordially co-operating with him.

The general effect of the first judicious management of patients is that it becomes practicable to examine their whole condition carefully, and to decide on the best plan of medical treatment. Of the medical or direct treatment of the patient, it is not the particular object of this work to speak. The collected opinions of the majority of medical superintendents of England, published a few years ago,* proved that experience had led nearly all of them to precisely similar conclusions respecting merely medical means. According to their united testimony, these means, really admissible in cases of insanity, are few and simple, deriving their chief efficacy from timely application. Venesection, formerly practised indiscriminately at "spring and fall," is almost universally proscribed, whilst the advantages of the local detraction of blood are acknowledged to be frequently very great; calomel

* Further Report of the Commissioners in Lunacy, 1847.

and antimony, once universally administered, are found to be but of occasional service ; and sedatives, although highly efficacious in certain cases, are often of no effect, and are sometimes hurtful. Emetics are seldom admissible. Aperient medicines are often required, and even purgatives ; although the latter are assuredly often abused. Baths, warm and tepid, and the shower-bath, tepid or cold, and variously modified, are useful in a great number of instances ; and the douche, although more severe than the shower-bath, is very seldom productive of peculiar benefit. The cold-bath is rarely employed ; but cold applications to the head, whilst the feet, or half, or the whole of the body are placed in warm water, are much used, and generally with advantage. Cold water poured upon the head is sometimes of signal service ; and patients will resort to this mode of relief of their own accord. The full use of the shower-bath can only be cautiously obtained by repeating the shower at short intervals (in a bath supplied by a cistern), and until decided prostration ensues. Employed in the ordinary manner, its effects are rather exciting than depressing. Blisters are occasionally useful ; setons and moxas seldom or never. Generally speaking, whatever reduces the strength of the patient acts unfavourably on the malady ; and the superintendents of asylums are unanimous in maintaining that the usual treatment must be tonic and generous, and the diet of the insane liberal and nutritious. Bodily exercise in the open air cannot be estimated too highly; the same may be said of occupation, not too early resorted to. The use of whirling-chairs, baths of surprise, violent affusions over the body, prolonged immersion in water, and all similar devices, are universally condemned; and speaking generally, the virtues of a long list of articles selected from the pharmacopœia, appear to be most confidently recounted by those who have had the fewest opportunities of putting them carefully to the test in large institutions.

These general practical views accord with my own experience. Bleeding, and the administration of strong purgatives, in the commencement of a maniacal attack, have usually appeared to me to be detrimental to the patient; and there are many recent cases in which sedatives, pushed to any extent, are at least useless. A combination of antimony with a sedative is sometimes more efficacious; but the depressing effects of antimony are too often only accompanied with temporary advantage. It is scarcely possible to predicate which of the several sedatives will have the best effect in any particular case; and the chief benefit of any of them has always seemed to me to be most conspicuous in chronic or recurrent cases; and far more remarkable in melancholia than in mania.

From the use of digitalis, once spoken of as a kind of specific, I never saw any advantage derived: the action of the heart becomes lowered, and the patient becomes faint or sick, but the cerebral excitement is not subdued by this medicine. Of violent emetics, repeatedly administered, and of strong stimulants, among the rest of wine, given to the extent of producing intoxication, methods which have been practised and praised, it is unnecessary to say more than that they appear to be the mere despair of medicine. Of calomel and other mercurial medicines I cannot speak favourably: their occasional use is undeniable; but a perseverance in their administration, except when indicated by the manifest presence of some bodily complication, is, I am convinced, useless, and sometimes mischievous. In the stage of recent excitement, blisters and all forms of counter-irritation prove generally unserviceable. The shower-bath, or the cold affusion on the head, variously combined with the warm-bath, the hip-bath, or the pediluvium, are as generally useful; and the local application of leeches, to the forehead, or behind the ears, or in many cases, in female patients, to the pubes or sacrum, are doubtless eminently serviceable; even in acute and recent cases.

It is always desirable to keep in view that the preternatural excitement of a patient affected with acute mania, his violent action, and his loud voice, are not indications of strength; and that the more violent the symptoms, the greater is the danger of sudden prostration and death. In young persons, maniacal symptoms are not unfrequently the first in the train of those belonging to pulmonary disease; of which the ordinary symptoms are long masked. In old persons an outbreak of mania is often the mere precursor of general decline and of death.

In chronic mania, except in the recurrent paroxysms incidental to every case, although very various in character, frequency, and intensity, in different cases, mere medical treatment is scarcely called for; except that each returning paroxysm requires to be met by treatment on the same principles as that of an incipient attack. The long intervals, during which the patients recover, in each case, more or less of perfect mind, afford opportunities for the application of all the methods of influencing the patient which belong to the non-restraint system. These impart to the patient his permanent character; modify his whole life; secure innumerable comforts to him; and win his grateful attachment.

Melancholia, when not the immediate result of powerful moral causes, is usually associated with more manifest bodily ailment than is generally detected in cases of mania; and clearer indications of treatment are frequently thus afforded. Among the general means commonly applicable are leeches, applied in small numbers and repeatedly, behind the ears, or to the epigastrium or other locality in which disorder is concluded to exist, followed by small blisters. Medicines which promote the action of the liver and digestive organs are also commonly required, and prove useful. Warm bathing and the shower bath, exercise, generous diet, and sedatives, are serviceable in almost all these cases. It often happens that this form of malady is associated with disease of the heart, or of the liver, or of some portion of the intestinal tract, or of the uterus; and occasionally, as in mania, the mental symptoms precede phthisis pulmonalis; usually, I think, in persons of middle or more advanced life. Each complication is of course to be considered.

The form of malady called general paralysis, and which, from its invariable association with mental impairment, might better be called the paralysis of the insane, presents, it is to be feared, few indications for confident medical treatment. Commencing with imperfect action in the muscles moving the lips, and in those connected with speech, and gradually invading all the voluntary muscles, and associated in almost every case with exaltation of mind and childish hopes and schemes, it appears to originate in a general affection of the brain, scarcely indicated after death by more than greater softness or greater firmness, general or partial, of the cerebral substance, and by ventricles full of serum, combined merely with other appearances common to all chronic cases of mental malady : and it leaves the practitioner, after the longest reflection, ignorant of its primary nature, and helpless as to its cure. Symptoms of more than usual excitement, occasionally recurring, are met and relieved by ordinary methods. Mercurial medicines, and powerful counter - irritants, are employed to suspend its course ; but as far as my own observation of such cases, not very limited, has taught me, absolutely without success. But the general treatment of these curious cases comprehends some of the most valuable resources of the non-restraint system ; productive of much comfort, and of many alleviations of incurable disease.

In the complications of mental disorder with epilepsy, all the ordinary resources of treatment are employed with more or less assiduity, according to the expectation in which the practitioner indulges of their being beneficial. Moderate local bleeding, a well ordered diet and carefully regulated bowels, at least produce frequent alleviation in this almost hopeless form of malady. The effect of more powerful remedies, administered as specifics, appears more than doubtful. Each seems, when first given, to afford relief ; but the virtues of all are found transient. The remarkable suspension of the attacks in some cases, and which arises from natural causes not at all understood, sometimes imparts what appears to be legitimate credit to any medicine which has been latest given.   Setons, moxas, and all violent counter-irritants, are, I fear, merely tormenting to the patient.   In these cases, and perhaps it may be added in all cases of mental disorder, the regular life led by patients in asylums is to a great extent remedial ; the diet and exercise contributing to physical improvement, and the absence of all ordinary causes of violent emotions keeping the brain in a tranquil condition, favourable to the recovery of healthy mental action.   For these reasons, a residence in a well-ordered asylum deserves to be ranked, in relation to a majority of cases of insanity, among the most efficacious parts of direct treatment.

Young and sanguine practitioners usually feel dissatisfied with candid statements of the possible inefficacy of medicines, resulting from experience ; and probably no physician undertakes the charge of an asylum without the pleasing belief that many of the cases considered incurable will recover with the aid of energetic treatment. It is to be regretted that this belief generally yields to repeated disappointments ; that chronic diseased conditions of the brain, reasonably presumed to exist, resist treatment adopted on what appear to be legitimate and reasonable grounds ; that some of the cases apparently not much removed from sanity never improve; and that others, which appeared the most unpromising, recover without our being able to explain the favourable termination. But there is still no reason to abandon the hope that fresh resources will some day be possessed by the practitioner; and that the real nature of the changes taking place in the brain may be better understood; and greater success attend medical treatment.

In determining on the course to be adopted in any case, a prudent practitioner will always first carefully inquire into the existence of any bodily ailment which can by possibility act on the brain; and it is a well established fact that the removal of such bodily ailment is often the precursor of mental amendment and restoration. In a great number of cases of mania and melancholia in female patients this is daily observed; and although the results may not be so certain or so general in forms of bodily disorder incidental to both males and females, still the examples of recovery under treatment directed to bodily disease are sufficiently numerous to encourage the practitioner. In too many instances, no such indications are offered for his guidance.

Such remarkable examples of recovery now and then occur, even after years of continued or of recurrent mental disorder, as to give some encouragement to the physician in cases apparently beyond hope. Some instances of this kind occurred at Hanwell, after seventeen or even twenty years of mental malady. These cases can, of course, only be regarded as exceptional; and they rather add to the obscurity of the pathology of mental disorders than to our confidence in remedies. They illustrate, however, the duty of still attending to the well-doing of the insane, however long afflicted. Practitioners familiar with insanity have probably all occasionally met with instances in which the patient, after a long attack of mania, has sunk into what appeared incurable dementia, remaining silent, and wholly apathetic for a great length of time; and yet in whom, when a local disease has supervened, attended with inflammation and pain, there has been a sudden revival of energy and of maniacal excitement, with recovery of voice and activity; but all subsiding with the subsidence of the local affection. These curious circumstances are naturally suggestive of a desire to produce similar but more permanent results by imitating these diseased local conditions; and to this end counter-irritants would also appear to be the best adapted. This method has accordingly been employed in some cases with striking effects, but often, also, with none; although in recurrent cases of mania, the external employment of the unguentum antimonii potassio - tartratis, and, in other cases, of blisters, is undoubtedly often useful. In cases of melancholia, blisters appear to be more efficacious.

There will soon be accumulated, I believe, in many asylums, very singular proofs of the general benefit of a tonic and nutritive plan of treatment in most of the forms of chronic insanity, and in all cases attended with obvious debility, in consequence of the recent extensive introduction of the use of the cod-liver oil into practice. The effects are scarcely more gratifying than the principle is important.

If the limitation of the direct therapeutical means applicable to mental disorders is so unsatisfactory, it is to be ascribed to the extreme obscurity in which the origin of cerebral disturbance is involved, and to the narrowness of our knowledge of the mental functions of the brain. In a great majority of cases of mania and melancholia, the condition of the brain in the commencement of the malady is entirely unknown; all conjecture about it is vague, and dissection reveals nothing. In older cases, the appearances found after death are the consequences of an anterior disturbance, of the nature of which we cannot always form a reasonable conjecture. In cases in which we are justified in concluding that a vitiated condition of the blood is the immediate cause of the disturbance of the brain, and in others in which plethora, or inanition and debility, are the evident causes, our indications of treatment are clearer. But even in these cases, as in all others, we speak of increased or diminished nervous energy as manifested in certain results, the nature of which is dimly comprehended by the most diligent mental physiologist. Although, in all probability, an exact knowledge of the nature of the nervous energy, and of the causes of its irregularities, may never be attainable, there is reason to hope that the zeal with which mental physiology is now cultivated, and the careful observations to which the brain is subjected, will eventually throw more light on the structure and offices of many parts of the nervous system, and lead to results of great importance to medicine and to mankind. To confess our present ignorance is merely to acknowledge that our science is not yet brought to perfection; and to be scrupulous in interfering with functions of great importance, disturbed in a manner unintelligible to us, is only consistent with the rational and cautious character of modern medicine. All practitioners in medicine whose experience extends, as my own does, to more than thirty years, must have observed, even within that short period, a striking change in the extent to which ordinary means, formerly considered remedial, and even indispensable, are employed. Large and frequent bleedings, once so common as almost to be universal, are now nearly unknown. Violent purgative medicines, and the excessive employment of mercury, by which rude attempts were made to force the performance of languid functions, have been desisted from in all climates where scientific practice prevails ; and it is admitted that the restoration of the general powers of the system is a more successful way to repair partial irregularities of action. These therapeutical changes, already still less general in country practice and in the English schools of medicine than they will assuredly become, are, doubtless, favourable to the health, comfort, and longevity of mankind. As the knowledge of diseases, and of the laws of health and life, become more and more attended to, the rashness of trusting to drugs alone will become more and more generally perceived ; and attempts to prevent the various physical afflictions to which human beings are subject will become steadier, more widely and scientifically entered upon, and more conspicuous in their results. The physician whose practice is especially directed to diseases of the brain and nerves has no reason to be dissatisfied if such views already influence the minds of those whom careful observation has led to conclusions which daily experience confirms. He need not be ashamed to acknowledge, with regard to mental phenomena, what has been expressed by one of the most scientific cultivators of physiology in our day, when avowing the impossibility of knowing in what the difference consists between the condition of the nervous system during sleep and when we are awake, that "neither our unassisted vision, nor the microscope, nor chemical analysis, nor any analogy, nor any other means at our disposal, enable us to form any kind of notion as to the actual changes in the brain or spinal cord on which any other nervous phenomena depend."*

In a region so obscure, to be cautious is to be wise, and presumptuous steps are but the steps of folly. The physician's office is assuming, in these times, a higher character in proportion as he ceases to be a mere prescriber of medicines, and acts as the guardian or conservator of public and of private health; studious of all agencies that influence the body and the mind, and which, affecting individual comfort and longevity, act widely on societies of human beings. Changes are gradually taking place even in special walks of medical practice in conformity to the enlightened principles by which the exertions of the officers of general health are directed; and these principles find an application, and are strikingly illustrated, in the modern asylums and modern treatment of the insane. Obscurity may yet hang over the origin of mental derangement; the explanation of sudden recoveries may continue difficult; the alterations incidental to portions of nervous matter may baffle investigation, and the possible varieties in the condition of the

* Psychological Inquiries. In a Series of Essays. By Sir Benjamin Brodie, Bart., 1854.

blood, often apparently associated with mental disturbance, may be yet unknown, or incapable of satisfactory elucidation; but general means have been revealed to men of science conducing to important modifications and ameliorations of mental malady. Improved diet, lodging, and clothing, greater personal cleanliness, and general sanitary regulations, have produced undeniably advantageous effects on the health and the duration of life on the insane. Frost-bite, mortification of the extremities, scorbutus, formerly prevalent and fatal in asylums, are now scarcely ever met with; dysenteries and severe diarrhœa, in former days the general accompaniments of insanity, are now not more prevalent in asylums than among the general population. Even cholera, which, in 1832, destroyed in some asylums one-third of the patients, has passed over the best regulated of them, in its subsequent visitations, marked only by a sudden increase of cases of severe diarrhœa, and with scarcely one fatal result. An equally striking diminution of the mortality in asylums has been observable since the establishment of the non-restraint system. Twenty years ago, the deaths in the licensed private houses near London were about 14 per cent., and in some other asylums more.* They have been, in some years

---

* Statistics of Insanity. By John Thurnam, M.D., Medical Superintendent of the Wilts County Asylum. Published 1845.

since that date, not more than 6 or 7 per cent. in the well regulated county asylums for insane paupers.

By far the greater number of agents which are found to be eventually remedial in insanity, are indirect in their operation, gradually influencing the mind itself. To all these the physician who wishes to maintain the non-restraint system must constantly and earnestly direct his attention. Under the ancient plan of treatment, medical means were often inapplicable, or not applied, and were sometimes used more for punishment and subjugation than as remedies for physical causes of malady. The resort to instruments of mechanical coercion was inconsistent alike with any medical consideration of the various forms of mental disease, and their causes, as it was with attention to the numerous auxiliary or moral means of cure which are so greatly relied upon where the ancient methods of control have ceased to be employed.

One of the chief of the indirect remedial means, because comprehending many means in one, is a cheerful, well-arranged building, in a well-selected situation, with spacious grounds for husbandry, and gardening, and exercise. The new asylums of England, as those of Derbyshire, Warwickshire, Wiltshire, Worcestershire, Hampshire, those of Coton-Hill, near Stafford, of Clifton, near York, of Manchester, erected near Cheadle, and of Prestwich, for a part of Lancashire, and also, it may justly be added,

G

a few of the asylums of older construction, as that of Northampton and of Staffordshire, and also that of Hanwell, for Middlesex—not surpassed in convenience, although greatly surpassed in size by the newer Middlesex asylum at Colney-Hatch—present, in various forms and degrees, examples of arrangements combining almost everything that benevolence can desire with all that the most cautious and experienced judgment demands: the old prison-air has departed, and asylums have really become, what Esquirol called them, instruments of cure.   Doors opening into gardens; flowers blooming round the windows; wide and light galleries; windows commanding agreeable views; sitting-rooms and bed-rooms, where neither bars, nor guards, nor heavy locks and keys are seen or required; convenient furniture; cleanliness everywhere; good bedding; baths and lavatories of the best construction; provision for warmth in winter, and for coolness and shade in summer; and every addition that can aid or protect the feeble, and benefit the sick, by day or by night, affording alleviation, and comfort, and rest for all the forms of pain and sorrow, present themselves in these noble institutions to the eye of the most careless observer, and afford a deeper satisfaction to those who know the effect of all these things on the patients than the contemplation of the grandeur of temples or of palaces.

Yet in such asylums the means of security are not omitted; they are even abundant, but never obtrusive. Well-devised doors and windows; knives of which the edges are so contrived as to prevent the infliction of serious or sudden injury; fire-guards, where most needed; the absence of all obvious or suggestive means of suicide; and the fitting up of a few padded rooms, neither dark, nor gloomy, nor unventilated, constitute the chief parts of the apparatus of safety required. Instead of the various galling restraints formerly considered necessary by day and by night, dresses are carefully adapted for such patients as are inclined to undress themselves, or to tear their clothes to pieces; dresses of substantial texture, and fastened by small locks instead of buttons. For those who cannot sleep, or to whom it is irksome to lie down, warm clothing is provided for the body and feet; and they are thus not deprived of their only relief, that of walking in their rooms in the night until weariness succeeds to nervous excitement, and repose to both. The general arrangements are such as facilitate a classification suited to the emergencies of difficult cases; providing for the quiet of such of the patients as are convalescent or improving, or, although incurable, are orderly, tranquil, and disposed to be industrious. Such arrangements include workrooms and work-shops of various kinds; as well as various modes of recreation, within doors and without, for the winter evenings and the summer days: books, drawings, musical instruments, chess, backgammon, billiards, swings, rocking-horses, cricket, bowls, ball-playing, kite-flying, &c. Some of the county asylums comprehend schools for the younger patients, and even for the older who wish to learn to read and write, and draw ; or to whom geography and an acquaintance with some parts of natural history afford pleasure.

A few years before the time when the use of mechanical restraints was discontinued at Hanwell, the ameliorations effected in the treatment of the insane by Esquirol, Pariset, Falret, and other French physicians, who, following Pinel, reprobated the abuse of chains and strait-waistcoats, enabled them to venture, without any inconvenience, on introducing even some of the gaieties of life among their patients—chiefly, however, among patients of the educated classes ; and the same attempt appears to have been made with equal success by Dr. Browne, at the asylum of Dumfries. About the same time, in many private asylums, the more tranquil patients were gradually permitted to enjoy the benefit of associating with the sane persons of the family ; the chief difficulty in effecting which arose from the unavoidable irritation now and then existing in the minds of the patients, either from having been put in restraints themselves, or from having seen restraints violently imposed on others. At that time, the precautions appropriate to a prison could not entirely be dispensed with; and the outcries of the secluded and chained occasionally penetrated to the parlour, and banished composure and confidence. Not even in the best private institutions, at that time, could the patients enjoy the perfect calmness arising from the certainty that, among those not present at the evening assembly, there was not one fastened to the wall of his room, or his bedstead; and from the conviction that it was better for those absent not to be exposed just then to social excitements. The extension of such occasional pleasures to a large majority of the patients in the largest asylums, and to patients of the ruder classes, seems to have only been attempted when the old instruments of coercion were rapidly disappearing from sight.

The non-restraint system was not yet quite established, although it was in active progress, at Hanwell, when (in August 1839) the attempt was made, on the female side of the asylum, with the very active co-operation of Miss Powell (now Mrs. Bowden), the young and zealous matron in that important period in the history of that institution, to introduce some of the livelier scenes of social life among the patients; and one of those large assemblages, or evening parties, took place which have since become so general, and which form no unimportant article of therapeutic application. On these occasions, the minds of the patients are necessarily animated by expectation, and by all the preparations for the party, such as the decoration of rooms, the devising of dress, &c. When the evening of the day comes, they are delighted by meeting all the attendants, all the officers, and several visitors; in whose presence they dance, and manifest much gaiety; yet controlling themselves in a very remarkable manner. They are supplied with tea, coffee, and refreshing fruits; and the male patients have an excellent supper. The music of a domestic band, partly composed of patients and partly of attendants, contributes to their free and perfectly harmless enjoyment. Some of them are easily persuaded to exhibit any peculiar accomplishment they possess, and play the violin or piano, or sing, or recite, or dance a hornpipe. All this is now so conducted as to exclude any anxiety on the part of the officers: the male and female patients are even allowed to meet at these domestic festivals; and, it is said, without any inconvenience being incurred. This would not have been prudent in the earlier attempts, when many patients were present who had often been exasperated by coercion; and there were, not unfrequently, disturbing outbreaks, now nearly if not quite unknown. The superintendents of asylums should, above all things, regard these

entertainments as remedial; which they truly may
be made. The enlivening effect of them begins
several days before the party takes place, and
continues for several days afterward. When the
evening commences, it is apparent that even the
patients of the pauper class feel, perhaps for the
first time in their lives, the pleasant animation
of mingling in a social manner with their neighbours. Those who have not yet become wholly
free from occasional paroxysms of violence restrain
themselves at least for the occasion. The convalescent wear an expression of the most serene
satisfaction; and a smile, seldom seen before, plays
on the countenance of the melancholic. These are
but outward expressions of mental states thus
induced, and which are approaches to recovery.
When the hour of separation arrives, all depart in
order, perhaps following the musicians; and the
cordial " good-nights" are touching to all to whom
the welfare of the patients is dear. From these
meetings more friendly feelings spring up between
the attendants and the patients, and between all
and the officers. The patients perceive that they are
cared for. The attendants learn the luxury of
doing good; and appreciate the notice and approbation of the officers, who observe their attentions.
And these impressions, repeatedly made, are found
to exercise so great an influence over the establishments for insane persons, that a special apartment

for recreation, called an entertainment-room, now constitutes a part of almost every asylum lately erected in England.

Such cheerful scenes, and such happy results, can only be realized in asylums in which the hideous features of restraint are unknown. If a female patient has been ill-treated, and after a scuffle in which caps have been destroyed and hair torn from the head, has been put into restraint by angry nurses, she will disdain to dance with those nurses, and despise their holiday smiles and attentions, as mere proofs of hypocrisy. If a male patient has been roughly treated by attendants, abused, struck, garotted, or put into a strait-waistcoat by them, he will probably quarrel with them, or knock one of them down, before the evening is over. But where restraints and violence are alike unknown, the patients and attendants have an equal enjoyment in the festivities, and look like affectionate friends; and if a violent man begins to demand the reason of his detention, he is soothed by a few words, and good humouredly postpones his representations until the next day; and then his discontent is forgotten.

In the best private asylums the patients are now often recreated by excursions in the neighbourhood, pic-nic parties, and visits to public exhibitions; care being taken both in the selection of patients and places. Evening parties, concerts, and dances are found to be practicable and useful. In some public asylums even dramatic performances are ventured upon.

All these things have been found to be compatible with the order and mild discipline necessary to be maintained in asylums. They imply a very complete system of vigilant superintendence, unostentatiously exercised by kind officers and attendants. In the old asylums they were unknown; and they never can be successfully engrafted on the old system; under which kind relations can scarcely subsist between the patients and those who have the care of them.

Among the minor attentions which operate favourably on the minds of patients, a supply of good Clothing is not to be forgotten. It is true that some of them prefer old and worn out garments to new ones, and are regardless of nicety of appearance; and that others delight in fantastic attire. Male patients will paint their hats, or twist them into various shapes; and women will dress their hair with ribbons and fragments of wool and coir and horse-hair; sometimes hoarding up strange finery of beads and lace, which is brought out with each returning accession of mental excitement. But these results of malady are consistent with a love of neatness and personal comfort in the majority of patients, or at least of a remaining sense of it, which the physician and the male and female officers under him should encourage. To poor creatures often placed in restraints or in coercion-chairs, dirtiness in every shape was unavoidable; and whilst these instruments were cherished, dirtiness was the rule of the house. A few patients were extravagantly indulged, and paraded before visitors; but the condition of the rest, as a patient himself once designated it to me, was "abject." I have seen pauper patients, formerly belonging to decent life, dressed in old military jackets, not so well dyed as to hide the original colour, and wearing scanty nether-garments of leather, bought by the thousand, at a rate so cheap as to delight the economical, who disregarded the want of fitting, or warmth, or comfort, or decency. The poor patients in the county asylums fully appreciate the comfort of a Sunday-dress; and the liberality which supplies a decent suit of clothes, or a neat gown and cap selected by the wearer, is by no means thrown away.

Inattention to clothing adapted to the season was one cause, although not the only cause, of scorbutus, so often prevailing in the old asylums, and of the occurrence of mortification of the extremities. Scorbutus, it has been observed, has nearly disappeared before the influence of good clothing and good diet; and mortification of the toes is scarcely ever met with, except in patients who have been kept long confined to a crib, in cold cells, and utterly neglected. If restraints are ever restored, both will be revived.

Another particular, which is of consequence to all persons, is especially so to insane persons in asylums: a supply of good and well-cooked Food, liberal in quantity and punctually served. The monotony of asylum-life is relieved by the certainty of comfortable meals, at regular hours. Pauper patients may be habituated to making some personal preparations for the dinner table, and patients of the higher class may readily be induced to dress for dinner. Insane people require a somewhat full diet; by which the body is nourished and the mind is satisfied. A good steward will take care that the food is always of good quality, and a good housekeeper will take care that it is well cooked. The manner in which the meals are conducted is of great importance; and here, as in every consideration respecting the daily life and habits of the insane, we are reminded of the indispensable necessity of having a staff of respectable and kind attendants; without which, neither the dress nor the diet of the patients will be properly attended to.

In visiting any asylum, it is always desirable to see the dinners, and as public asylums are now conducted, the sight is generally gratifying. The manner in which the various meals are prepared for the patients at Hanwell, the food itself, and its mode of distribution in the wards, are highly satisfactory; and those who have opportunities of observing the influence of these comfortable arrangements on the patients, well know how valuable they are. In the best private asylums the more reasonable patients often form an agreeable dinner-party of ladies and gentlemen; and every patient in the house is fed carefully and decently. There are still, I fear, some private asylums in which patients of higher rank enjoy no such attentions. Their whole dinner is taken to them on one plate; not always with a knife and fork; and a table-cloth, salt, &c., are considered superfluous. It is also to be apprehended that neither the quality nor the quantity of the food receive proper consideration. Either in private or public asylums, patients in restraints are inevitably and shockingly neglected in these particulars. A patient in a strait-waistcoat cannot feed himself; those patients who are in coercion-chairs usually tear their food to pieces and devour it like animals; those who are fastened down in bed are too often deprived of part of their food, and left also to suffer from thirst. An ambition has very recently sprung up in some of the largest asylums to exhibit nearly all the patients at once at the hour of dinner, in the large entertainment-room The advantage of this display is not by any means obvious; and, without new and especial precautions, this public exhibition may lead to forgetfulness or neglect of those who cannot traverse immense corridors, and ascend and descend staircases, and who must necessarily dine in the wards to which they belong. Everything that comforts or gratifies the patients is worthy of adoption, but, both as respects these large dinner assemblies, and the evening entertainments themselves, arrangements so recommended should be carefully distinguished from such as are merely ostentatious: still, ever keeping in view that the object of all arrangements in an asylum should be remedial, and that considerations of an inferior kind cannot worthily be entertained.

The order and cheerfulness of an asylum, the cleanliness, the good food, produce that habitual state of comfort and tranquillity in the majority of the patients, of which one effect is the quietness of the wards at night. In walking through the long galleries at Hanwell at late hours, and sometimes with medical visitors, nothing has seemed so impressive as the silence prevailing throughout. The screams and horrible sounds described in old institutions are either unknown, or, if ever unexpectedly heard, are attended to without an instant's delay; and thus lead to the removal of some real or imaginary cause. Generally, the only exception to the entire repose was that of wakeful patients talking to themselves; referring to the events of the past day, or to the recollected events of their earlier years—of youth, of childhood: and all without anger, and without expressions of distress. This calm state of so many insane persons was doubtless the result, in many, of exercise and occupation during the day ; and, in most of the rest, of their general state of comfort. To be well clothed, to have a comfortable bed, and sufficient good food every day may, of course, be considered as having peculiarly comforting effects on pauper patients, too long accustomed to scanty fare, and miserable lodging, and wretched clothing. They often come to the asylum half starved, and good food is not unfrequently of far more consequence to them than medicine of any kind. But the circumstances conducive to physical comfort are important to all patients ; and even the richer patient soon begins to have tranquil nights, when he lies down in an asylum where during the day he has suffered no privation or indignity, and where he hopes, also, to awake the next day in peace, and that the next day, and the next, will find him still surrounded by comforts. Among these, in every class, sufficient food, of good quality, is one of the chief importance. Indeed, its being supplied is in itself a proof that innumerable sources of satisfaction receive due attention.

To secure all these advantages, the physician must be able to command the services of a staff of kind and conscientious attendants trained by himself. If the attendants are accustomed to the sight of their patients in the humiliating condition of restraints, and allowed to impose restraints whenever a patient is wayward or irritable, for every irregular action, and for every violent word, they cannot be trained to treat the same patients with any show of respect, much less with any constant manifestation of humane regard. When the patient is tied up, all regard for him ceases. Attendants are generally persons of small education, and easily inflated by authority: they love to command rather than to persuade, and are too prone to consider their patients as poor lost creatures, whom they may drive about like sheep. Nothing can prevent the expression of these narrow sentiments in action but the vigilant superintendence of superior officers, acting under one head. For the real duties demanded of attendants are nearly incessant. The dresses of patients require frequent adjustment; the order to be preserved at the dinner-table calls for constant care; and, in the midst of many interruptions, all must be done quietly, and patiently, and gently. There must be constant attention, and even frequent interference, so delicately managed that the patients suspect no watching, and take no umbrage at the necessary care extended to them. By such a course of conduct the attendants acquire great control over the patients under their immediate charge, who soon begin to look upon them as their protectors to whom they can apply for any moderate indulgence, and appeal in every little trouble. Then, indeed, the true restraint is exercised over patients—the restraint of the feelings and the mind. Any display of anger, or any act of injustice, on the part of the attendant, and any gross neglect or insult, destroys this influence; and if such attendant can rush to a repository of strait-waistcoats and handcuffs by way of enforcing his authority, agitation and terror soon prevail in his ward, and the charm of kindness is broken and lost.

In the Returns made by the Superintendents of County Asylums to the Commissioners in Lunacy (*Eighth Report*, 1854), the brutalizing effect on the attendants themselves of being accustomed to resort to mechanical restraints is forcibly expressed by those who know both the old system and the new. This effect is strongly manifested by them in their demeanour to a patient, and which is usually productive of aversion at the first interview. Insane persons regard all strangers with suspicion, and observe them very narrowly. A kind expression of face, a friendly manner, and a gentle voice, has great influence over them; and they will often agree to do anything that is recommended by one whose possession of these qualities has prepossessed them agreeably. The attendant of the old asylums too often approaches a new patient roughly; looks upon him with the same kind of countenance with which he would regard a vicious horse that he had undertaken to subdue; is provided with various instruments of coercion, which he puts on if he receives the slightest provocation, and in the putting on of which he does not scruple to use any kind of violence to the feelings, or injury to the person of the patient, whom he conquers at length by brute force, and over whom he triumphs in a manner he makes no attempt to conceal.

One most material part of the non-restraint system, consequently, taken in its fullest signification, is the selection of proper attendants: and as in the former state of asylums most of the attendants were merely persons unfit for any other employment, their general character was fierce and presuming, and they were utterly untrustworthy; so, even in some of the largest asylums, one of the physician's greatest difficulties is to conduct the asylum with attendants chosen by the governors, or by officers who are very partially subjected to his authority, and indifferently affected to his plans of treatment; and it must be with grief that he oftentimes beholds his male patients subjected to the control of discharged servants, idle and dissipated mechanics, and other objectionable characters, to whom he would not himself have entrusted the care of valuable dogs. The frequent changes among the female attendants is also generally such

H

as to deprive the superintendent at any time of a
sufficient number possessing experience, or of any
one fit to be entrusted with the special treatment
of difficult cases. In both the male and female
departments, also, although minor faults are often
inconsiderately punished, the bad treatment of the
patients is not so promptly followed by expulsion as
the safety of the patients demands; and, generally,
the knowledge possessed by the attendants that
they are independent of the physician impedes him
in many ways, and makes it quite impossible that
he should carry out the complete system existing in
his mind.

The importance of this particular in the
government of asylums cannot be exaggerated.
The physician who justly understands the non-
restraint system well knows that the attendants are
his most essential instruments; that all his plans,
all his care, all his personal labour, must be counteracted, if he has not attendants who will observe
his rules, when he is not in the wards, as conscientiously as when he is present. No one can select
them for him, for no one can fully understand all
the qualities which his views require them to
possess. Unless, therefore, this privilege of choos-
ing them himself is accorded to him, and unless
his officers exercise a vigilant supervision over
them, as directed by himself, whatever good may

be done in any asylum, the governors must not flatter themselves that they are fully carrying out the non-restraint system.

Let it be considered what functions are entrusted to the attendants. First, the peculiar attentions described as practised on the admission of a new patient. A kind attendant leads the timid or distrustful stranger into the wards as into a home of refuge. An unkind attendant leads the new patient into the ward with no more consideration than he would lead an animal into its stall. Nearly all the details of the first treatment, already mentioned, and which are so influential on the patient's course in the asylum, must be confided to attendants. Many of the insane take their character from the attendant under whom they are placed; so that under one they become morose, sullen, and dangerous; under another tranquil and docile. The physician requires the agency of cheerful helpers, healthy and contented, of natural good disposition, and possessed of good sense. His government of them should be such as to preserve their cheerfulness, and health, and contentment. They are his instruments, and he should keep them finely tempered. They may often be considered, indeed, his best medicines; and they should be well chosen and well preserved. He confides the most confidential duties to them: he entrusts them with the happiness, by day and by night, of all the patients under their especial care. To control the violent, without anger; to soothe the irritable, without weak and foolish concessions; to cheer and comfort the depressed; to guard the imbecile and the impulsive, and to direct all—these are great duties to be demanded from such instruments; and no security for their proper performance is to be found except in the character of the attendants themselves, and in the manner in which they are themselves treated. If the physician has proper authority, and is worthy to possess it, he governs the attendants with equity, directs rather than reproves them, supports them in difficulty, and protects them by his regulations from being frequently exposed to danger. He is careful to afford them as many intervals of relaxation as possible, knowing that a loss of physical health must disqualify them for the delicate and trying tasks which they are expected to perform. In return, they obey him because they respect him. But all this is impracticable where the authority over them is divided, and due subordination to one head does not exist. It is in vain for boards and committees of asylums to attempt to substitute, for such good government, a clause of an Act of Parliament, or any formal obligation, signed by attendants, ill-selected by themselves.

The medical officers residing in the asylum can best appreciate the value of the services of the attendants, and understand how much a system of non-restraint is blended with the duties expected of them every hour. Insane persons are so generally excitable that the hasty passing through a ward by an irritable or angry officer, or a self-important and noisy committee-man, leaves traces of agitation for some time perceptible to those who know the patients. Even such imprudence is an infraction of the non-restraint system; the great principle of which is to exclude all hurtful excitement from a brain already disposed to excitement. On this principle it abolishes mechanical restraint : and also, on this principle it regulates every word, look, and action of all who come in contact with the insane. The operation of the principle must be universal to be complete. It must prevail from the unlocking of the bed-room doors in the morning to the hour of closing them for the night, and must even be active in its application to particular cases through all the anxious hours between the evening and morning. The melancholy must be cheerfully encouraged to get up, the feeble must be assisted, the occurrence of any new ailment noticed and attended to : the washing and dressing of the patients must be superintended ; their morning meal comfortable, and decently served ; those who desire it must be accompanied to chapel, and those who are employed in various occupations, placed still under kind guidance, distributed through the workshops and laundries, and gardens and grounds. That done, special attention is demanded for the more troublesome or the more helpless patients; to dressing them, and getting them out of doors; and the patients who are employed within doors and those who do not care to be employed must be taken out into the fields or large airing courts. All the dinner tables are superintended by the attendants, who are expected to attend kindly, to prevent occasions of quarrel, and to regulate everything. That meal concluded, the afternoon brings a return of exercises or occupations, the latter being proportioned to the patient's state, over which, from day to day, the attendants are required to be watchful, lest moderate labour, which is found widely remedial, should become a punishment or a distress. Not later than five o'clock, the work ceases, or ought to cease: then there should be tea for the patients; a short evening service in the chapel; and after some in-door or out-door amusements, according to the season, a plain supper for the men; and then all should begin to retire to clean beds in well-ventilated sleeping-rooms. And for all these details of every day the physician must rely mainly on the attendants; who, on their part, must be ever watchful and active, preventing accidents, and guarding against outbreaks of violence; making themselves to a great extent the companions of their patients, helping to amuse and cheer them, to soothe and direct them ; omitting no observation of their appearance, manners, and language ; reporting their wants and wishes to the physician, and not overlooking indications of amendment.   And all this they are required to do with cheerfulness, and with a perfect command of temper.   Such are the duties required of attendants in an asylum conducted on the non-restraint principle.   Such, kindly and efficiently performed, day after day, are in fact the all-powerful substitutes for mechanical restraints. It is unnecessary, then, to say more on the importance of their selection, or of its being left to the physician.

I cannot dismiss this portion of my subject without saying, that many years' experience of public institutions, including my residence in the Hanwell asylum, has convinced me that it is not difficult to obtain and preserve good attendants, male and female, in asylums, or good nurses in the infirmaries of asylums, if they are chosen with even moderate discretion, and if they are kindly and justly governed.   Their duties are fatiguing, depressing, often repulsive ; and they require support and cheerful encouragement for their proper performance of them.   If, instead of this, they are governed unkindly and tyrannically ; if no fault is overlooked ; if the entrance of the male or female officers into the wards is always the preface to cold and discouraging remarks, or to hasty rebukes, the spirits of the attendants sink. If they are gentle in disposition, despondency and tears, and inaction and neglect, are the consequences: if they are more spirited, the result is insubordination and anger, and harsh treatment of the patients under their charge. The defects of government in these particulars are generally most prevalent on the female side of asylums; where severe regulations, including restrictions as to leave of absence and reasonable holiday, are often unfavourable both to the bodily and mental health of the attendants, who are yet expected to manifest an active solicitude for the bodily and mental health of their patients ; and, generally, to exhibit all the cardinal virtues. This is the mere vice of domestic servitude transferred to public institutions.

An important change was introduced into asylums a few years before the era of the abolition of mechanical restraints, but still only partially and imperfectly ; its perfect accomplishment only proving practicable in proportion as that great measure began to show its general effects on the mind of the lunatic. This was the introduction of regular religious observances, and of all the consolations of religion, among the inmates of asylums. The attempt was at first discountenanced in many such institutions ; even derided. Experience

has proved that a kind and judicious chaplain may
be a valuable auxiliary to the physician. But the
introduction of regular services in a chapel before
the old violent methods of coercion were given up
and forgotten, was attended with peculiar anxieties.
Sunday was represented as being always a day of
agitation. Sudden interruptions of the clergyman,
and incidents of a very disturbing character were,
indeed, common in the chapel. These seemed
always to arise among patients who had recently
been kept in restraints; as if during the service
their excited minds had brooded over their past
sufferings or wrongs, until they could control their
feelings no longer, and therefore' broke out into
loud and passionate exclamations, or made a sudden
rush at the physician, or at the clergyman himself.
When, from the entire absence of mechanical
restraints, and the introduction of all the improvements belonging to the non-restraint system,
the wards had assumed a character of habitual
tranquillity, and the patients were, as a part of the
system, brought to chapel decently and neatly
dressed, and were supplied with prayer-books, and
assisted by attendants sitting among them, the
chapels of the asylums became, what they now
are, places of perfect quietness and order, exercising the best effects on the patients, and deeply
interesting to all who are devoutly and humbly

disposed; whilst, throughout the wards, Sunday is peculiarly a day of calmness and rest.

By these various appliances, some of them singly of small significance, and perhaps almost wearisome in detail, but conjoined forming a complete system directed to one object, the whole constitution of an asylum, and the transactions and incidents of every day, are made remedial. Everything done by every officer, and every word spoken by the sane to the insane, is in conformity to one plan, directed by a chief physician, carried out in all its details by efficient and faithful officers, and having for its sole object the happiness of the patients, the relief or cure of all the griefs and troubles of the heart, and the restoration of composure and power to the mind. These, in their union, constitute the system of managing the insane without mechanical restraints.

From the journals of any asylum in which such principles are really acted upon, innumerable cases might now be cited illustrative of their beneficial operation. Patients are doubtless still received into such institutions from places into which no such principles have yet penetrated; and their improved condition must continually illustrate the advantages of an improved treatment. But the deep anxiety felt by the earlier practisers of non-restraint can scarcely now be imagined by superintendents who have the cheering light of the experience of their predecessors to guide them. Pinel found that when the clanking of chains ceased, the patients became calm. Charlesworth and Hill found that when mechanical restraints were destroyed, unexpected and vast improvement followed in the lunatics under their charge. But the first years of the non-restraint system at Hanwell were also full of anxieties; although soon almost every week furnished some examples of amendment which afforded encouragement, and did not suffer hope to die.

Of these, a few may be quoted, notwithstanding that, happily, similar examples have now become more or less familiar in all the large asylums of England. On the female side of the house, where the greatest daily amount of excitement and refractoriness was to be met and managed, the cases of recent insanity in young women, and especially the cases of puerperal insanity, and those arising from lactation, were perhaps the first to attract particular notice in reference to the new system. Anywhere but where restraints are indiscriminately employed, such cases would seem the likeliest to be regarded with interest and compassion, and to be treated with gentleness. But as they are usually attended with a great degree of excitement, and with a lively propensity to every kind of mischief, and consequently occasion much trouble, these cases had become more especially and constantly subjected to severe coercion.

In successive years, numerous cases of this kind were admitted at Hanwell. In 1844, a young woman, then unmarried, who had been in the asylum two years before, and in a state of mania, and who recovered from that attack within twelve months from its commencement, returned to us, having had a relapse, whilst nursing an infant ten months old. Cases of mania from protracted nursing, together with deficient nourishment, are not, it is well known, unfrequent; and they usually improve and recover when these causes of weakness and exhaustion are removed. This patient was pale, emaciated, restless, and disposed to destroy her clothes. Her pulse was 120, and feeble; the tongue clean, the head cool. Her mind was confused; and she talked rapidly and incoherently. Unfortunately, she had been first taken to a private asylum, where restraints were in ordinary use, and the causes of the insanity, and all medical treatment, as usual, neglected. As soon as she arrived there, she had one leg fastened by a chain to the bedstead by night; and in the daytime she wore a strait-waistcoat, and was fastened by the leg to a grating. Nobody, she told us, used to come near her; and she was left to cry from vexation and the pain caused by the strait-waistcoat. As soon as this patient was admitted at Hanwell, she was subjected to the *non*-restraint treatment; that is, she not only was freed from the strait-waistcoat, and unfastened by a chain in the night or during the day, but she was carefully and specially attended to; good and sufficient food was supplied to her; she was kindly waited upon; warm baths were administered, and occasional sedatives. From the first day of her admission she began to recover. For a month afterward the maniacal state continued, but the patient was satisfied and good-humoured. In six weeks she had made considerable progress towards recovery, and her pulse had subsided to 88. Her appetite was excellent, and she improved greatly in appearance. Within three months from her admission she left the asylum quite well.

About the same time, another case, more strictly puerperal, was brought to the asylum. A young married woman (ætat 23) was admitted two months after confinement. When in childbed, a fire broke out in a neighbouring house. She was extremely alarmed; and mania ensued. She was taken to one of the licensed private asylums near London: there this poor delicate woman was put into a strait-waistcoat, and wore iron handcuffs by day, and was fastened to the bedstead by night. Her peculiar condition, her recent fright and agitation, were alike disregarded; and her physical state apparently quite neglected. She was troublesome, not dangerous, but still subjected to coarse restraint. She was maniacal, and her cure was trusted to leathern straps and manacles of iron. She came to the Hanwell asylum in a strait-waistcoat; which was immediately taken off. When visited by the medical officers, her appearance was found to be sickly, and her head excessively hot; the uterine functions were suspended; her tongue was red; her pulse 120, and very feeble. She was timid, agitated, and cried much; and spoke affectionately of her husband. Her slender wrist was marked with restraints. She was immediately soothed by the kindest attentions; cold applications were applied to the scalp, and were very grateful to her; a little medicine was given; and she speedily began to regain composure and to feel some confidence in those about her. This case occurred at the time of the annual course of clinical lectures and visits; and it was watched from week to week, with much interest, by the students. In about ten days, convalescence had fairly commenced; and she was well enough to see her husband. She then became employed in the fancy-work room; and in a month she left us, quite well. Five months afterward, she came to see her friends at the asylum: she remained perfectly well; but the mark of the handcuffs remained also.

Instances occurred occasionally among the young women brought to the asylum, affected with puerperal insanity, of such as were stupid and ferocious, turning fiercely and dangerously on those around them. These patients had generally been fastened down, and allowed to lie neglected and miserable on wet straw. Their recovery under careful and gentle treatment was, however, gradual and remarkable. In a few days some intelligence appeared in the countenance; and by degrees every sign of satisfaction and confidence. Many cases of this kind are rescued by the non-restraint treatment from incurable imbecility and death.

On Christmas-day, in the year 1850, having just been round the wards at the dinner hour, and witnessed the general cheerfulness of the house, and the pleasure derived by the patients from the good English fare provided for them, I found, on approaching the reception-room on the female side, an unexpected confusion and agitation, and several nurses assembled, and evidently disturbed by some new occurrence of a different character. They reported that a patient, a married woman (about twenty-four years of age), had just been brought to the asylum in a state of violent excitement. The patient was labouring under acute mania. Of her history no account had been obtained from those who brought her. She had evidently been subdued by main force, and bound with great severity, and brought hastily and roughly to the asylum. Those who brought her immediately left her, as if glad to get away; not even staying to see the medical officers or matron. Everything seemed to add to the terror of this young woman. She made great resistance to being undressed, and to being placed in a warm bath. She was found to have several bruises ; and one ankle had already become ulcerated by leg-locks or some kind of bonds. Either her malady, or the treatment to which she had been subjected before admission, or both together, had inspired her with the dreadful idea that she was about to be burned alive ; and the strong resistance made by her to any thing attempted by the attendants was caused by her alarm and suspicion as to their intentions. In every one who approached her she seemed to behold an enemy, or an executioner.

It may readily be supposed that in a case of this kind, a stern reception, the continuance or the imposition of restraints, and a darkened room, would only have confirmed .the patient's fears, and have aggravated them to frenzy and despair, ending, in all probability, in death. Yet she was not in a state capable of receiving immediate consolation ; nor could she, all at once, be made to understand that she was surrounded by those whose intentions were friendly and kind. What her condition required was the temporary withdrawal of all the attendants, and consequent quiet; with time to recover some degree of composure. There was no more effectual way of procuring these advantages than by resorting to temporary seclusion, of which such a case well exemplified the good influence. When, therefore, not without difficulty, she was dressed after having had a warm bath, the attendants carried her, notwithstanding unavoidable struggles, into a clean apartment, not darkened, but having the window guarded, and of which all the walls were padded, and all the floor was a sort of bed, covered with a thick mattress. In a short time she was left there, but was frequently looked at during the day through the inspection-plate in the door. The tranquillity and the solitude appeared at first to surprise her. She got up, and walked about the room as if to examine it; then lay down again, and became quiet and composed. It was some hours before she became quite calm enough to take a little food, and by this time the appearance of the attendants scarcely seemed to alarm her. After three days' careful nursing and management she had quite gained confidence in them, and it was practicable to remove her to a bed in the infirmary. In a few weeks, by medical treatment, and the constant care of kind nurses, she recovered, without interruption, and without relapse.

About the same time, and whilst I still had the advantage of Dr. Hitchman's co-operation, to whom these cases were no less the especial objects of interest than to myself, another young and delicate woman was admitted—a widow, whom distress had rendered distracted. She was brought to the asylum unattended by any female, but very closely secured in *two* strait-waistcoats; her ankles were also carefully fastened together by a chain. On her arrival she was irritable, angry with everybody, suspicious of everybody, and seemed likely to prove for a time intractable.   When assured by Dr. Hitchman that the waistcoats and chain should be immediately taken off, and should not be put on again, she at first seemed to distrust these assurances. Finding that they were really to be carried into effect, she broke out into the liveliest expressions of joyful gratitude ; and from that time, although still for a while maniacal, and often excited, her confidence in those about her remained unshaken.   A gradual improvement took place, and in about three months she left the asylum perfectly rational, although still unable, without agitation and tears, to speak to us of the treatment she had suffered in one of the workhouses from which she had been brought to Hanwell.

Much excuse must be admitted for the exposure of the insane poor in workhouses to such severe treatment, ill supplied as those houses generally must be with better means of safety and control.   But the occurrence of such instances of restraint year after year, after all that has been done in county asylums,

strongly exemplifies the importance of communi-
cating to medical practitioners, both in town and
country, such a share of knowledge and experience,
as respects the treatment of insane people, as may
protect afflicted men and women from needless
pains and vexations, too well calculated to add to
the excitement of disease, and to render recovery
less probable. In this respect, much yet remains to
be done, both in London and in the provinces.

An officer living in an asylum, and really intimate with the insane, can scarcely fail to become
interested in persons who in the wreck of mind
retain often so many valuable feelings. Fear and
anger are not long the emotions they excite, but in
their stead sympathy and compassion. Soon after
my appointment to Hanwell I learned this lesson.
Among other patients admitted was a poor tailor's
wife; she had already been insane some months,
after a confinement, and, apparently, from want of
nourishment and comforts. She was a kind of mad
skeleton. Looking as if she might at any moment
drop down and die, she still danced, and sung, and
ran to and fro, and tore her clothes and all ordinary
bedding to rags. We had just begun to meet these
difficulties without restraints, and she was indulged
in some of her harmless fancies; supplied, among
other things, with useless remnants that she might
amuse herself with tearing them into shreds. Good
food was given to her, and porter. She became

stouter, and she became calmer; and soon she employed herself in making dresses instead of tearing them: and thus a happy recovery was commencing, when her poor husband came to see her. The sight of him, half-starved and half-clothed, distressed her, and caused a temporary relapse. She became depressed, wept bitterly, and lamented that her husband could not also come into Hanwell. These feelings were counteracted by the desire to go to her home, poor as that home was, and to comfort her husband, and share his poverty: and as soon as she was well enough her wish was complied with.

It was extremely touching, in these my early days of asylum life, when every day was eventful, and every event was instructive, to find that more tears began to be shed by the female patients on leaving the asylum than on entering it. Before going, several of them soon began to petition not only to be allowed to go into the matron's parlour, and the kitchens, store-rooms, and work-rooms in which they had been employed, and to take a kind and grateful leave of the officers; but also, as a particular favour, to visit the particular ward in which they had been placed on their first coming to the asylum—generally a refractory ward—where they would embrace the nurses and many of the poor patients, and with affectionate expressions, and sobs, and broken words, would promise to

come and see them again if they could.   These
promises were often performed.   Witnessing these
scenes, not without emotion, and reviewing them
at the quiet close of each busy and anxious
day, I began to feel assured that the system we
were pursuing, however difficult, could not be
wrong.   When my first attempts to convey clinical
instruction in the asylum were made, the pupils
attending the visits and lectures now and then
derived most valuable information from the opportunities they had of seeing newly admitted cases.
The evidence thus afforded to them of what might
be done by the simple removal of exciting restraints
was irresistible.   During the first course of this
kind, in May, 1842, a remarkably fine looking
young woman (æt. 20) was brought to the asylum,
wearing a strait-waistcoat very tightly put on.
Her face was flushed; her eyes were animated;
she was extremely noisy and excited; talked loudly,
and frequently sung; but was very irascible with
everybody who came near her.   It was observed
that both the wrists and ankles of this young
person were ulcerated, as if by having worn iron
handcuffs and leg-locks.   The strait-waistcoat was
taken off, and the patient being put into a warm
bath, ceased to be angry, and expressed her sense
of the relief in the liveliest terms.   Her cerebral
excitement had supervened on uterine irregularity;
and the treatment of the bodily disorder by leeches,

the warm bath, and gentle aperient medicines, combined with rest, tranquillity, and the general kindness of those about her, soon restored her to perfect health. But the mere discontinuance of the restraints, and the friendly reception given to her on admission, had a striking effect; and in two days afterward she was induced to do some needle-work in the matron's room; Miss Powell— the matron at that time—having taken the case, according to her frequent custom, under her special care. On the third day, the students being at the asylum, were allowed to see her there; two or three going into the room at a time. She was still considerably excited, and fancied the students were all her children: she was disposed to laugh loudly and long; but influenced by quiet words, and perfectly good-tempered. She complained, however, that before coming to Hanwell, she had worn "those infernal fetters" day and night for three weeks. This young woman recovered rapidly and entirely, when restraints were used no longer, and when she was regarded as a patient brought under our care to be cured of illness of body and disorder of mind. No doubt could exist in the minds of the observers of this case, that many such, neglected in many miserable asylums, passed on to chronic and incurable stages.

A case, indeed, had presented itself a few months before (M. F. admitted in January, 1842), in which death from such neglect appeared imminent. A young married woman (æt. 25) who had been insane eighteen months, and whose malady ensued on protracted nursing, probably together with semi-starvation, was brought to us tied up in complicated restraints, although she was greatly emaciated, and so feeble as literally to be unable to walk. Her wrists were wounded and her ankles ulcerated with the restraints she had worn; and her toes were in an actual state of mortification. She appeared frightened, and her expression of countenance was wild and haggard. Altogether she looked as if merely sent to the asylum to end her miserable life. She was, of course, at once liberated from her restraints; and with the great care bestowed upon her, she began in a few weeks to recover the power of moving about, and her general aspect became less wretched. For several weeks afterward she was wild, and disposed to be mischievous, although perfectly harmless. Good food, wine, liberty, fresh air, and the sense of having kind people about her, wrought wonderful effects. She became stout, healthy, and gradually quite reasonable. Two of her toes were lost; but her life was saved. She had a distinct recollection of the events of her illness; told us that for a length of time she had worn a strait-waistcoat in the day-time, her wrists being at the same time confined by iron handcuffs; and that at night both her hands and feet had been fastened to the bedstead. Eventually she left the asylum quite recovered.

At that time, some illustration or other of the contrasted effects of the old treatment and the new was continually to be met with in the wards. Young women, especially, were often brought to the asylum reported "furious;" their wrists and ankles marked or ulcerated with restraints. The effect of removing all these cruel instruments was always satisfactory. A disposition to violence might remain, and paroxysms recur, and suicidal tendencies linger in the thoughts for a time; but the patient was controlled by kindness, and life preserved by vigilance. Sometimes, in paroxysms of excitement, distressing images of force and terror long afterward recurred to the minds of these patients. In their calmer intervals they would relate the severities inflicted upon them; often, it seemed, by men, who were employed to overpower them, or throw them into a cold bath, or chain them. The lively gratitude of these patients to those who liberated them never died away; and the resulting calmness soon made it difficult to show the clinical pupil, in the extensive wards of Hanwell, an aggravated case of furious mania.

Gratifying results of the uniform plan of gentle treatment became, in the course of a few months, and more and more in successive years, visible in every ward of the asylum; and often of a character which excited deep emotion in those whose first attempts to effect such a change had been accompanied with frequent anxiety, and, now and then, with sorrow and even anguish, amidst misrepresentations and devices now not worth recording, and almost forgotten. Patients who when first received were silent or incoherent, miserable in attire, and whose wretchedness was only varied by occasional fits of passion, became neat in dress, orderly in habits, cheerful in countenance. Others, who came half starved, sickly, comfortless, and wholly irrational, became composed, healthy looking, active, and useful. Those even who came in a state of dangerous violence seemed soon to be acted upon by the character of the house, and gradually to become sensible of being surrounded by kind persons, who spoke to them as to reasonable creatures, expressed sorrow and not anger when they were unruly, and used glad and encouraging words when they were tractable and industrious. There were now and then, among the new admissions, young women on whom various terrors had had the effect of producing the profoundest melancholy, accompanied with an expression of dread. They were usually feeble, sickly, and appeared to be acquainted only with misery; they would not speak; they would scarcely take food; and they stood against the walls, their hands crossed over the bosom, the very personification of despair. Recovering gradually from this state, they would tell us that, even in that apparent torpor, they watched everything that was done, and were attentive to every observation that we made; and by degrees they understood us, and tried to rouse themselves. After recovery, promoted by medical means, and the shower bath, and good diet, and cheering and comforting words daily addressed to them, it was often as surprising as it was delightful to see them converted into cheerful hopeful creatures, full of health and spirits, and unfeignedly grateful to those who had been their friends in the asylum; and at length able to return to their families perfectly recovered in mind.

Nor was it in recent cases, nor in young persons alone, that the effects of a mitigated treatment were strongly manifested. Older patients, who had been for years subject to recurrent mania and melancholia, and sent in different attacks to different places of confinement, and worn into chronic irritation by repeated sufferings in such places, became, although more slowly, tractable and confiding under the new treatment. The paroxysms of the malady became shorter in several instances, and the violence of the paroxysms generally less. Some of these patients were disposed in time to talk in a friendly manner both with the officers and the attendants; and I several times derived instruction from their sorrowful experiences. From one female patient, forty-six years of age, and who had been for nearly twenty of these years liable to attacks of insanity, and whose strength and violence in the attacks had caused the strait-waistcoat to be had recourse to as soon as any warning deviation from her usual manner was observed, I learned, that when scarcely thirty years of age she lost her husband, and soon afterward a child to which she was much attached. Her husband had been the master of a vessel, and the widow kept an inn much resorted to by sea-faring persons of a respectable class. But her house still seemed desolate to her, and her continued grief led to negligence of her affairs. Embarrass-ments followed, and many disquietudes. She became absent and distracted in mind, often for-getting what she was about, sometimes sitting down at breakfast-time, and then only recollecting that she had not lighted any fire. The doors of her house were often left insecure by her, from forget-fulness, and her goods were stolen. At length she became too decidedly deranged to carry on her business, and her malady assumed the form of melancholia, alternating with maniacal excitement, and she was taken to one of the old asylums near London, then among the worst of its kind, but in

which the treatment of the patients is now so
humane and excellent that it would be unjust
even to name it in connection with this case.
The history of this patient, and the afflictions
which had caused her mind to give way, would
now receive attention in that and in all good
asylums. But the day had not arrived for such
kind sympathies, and on arriving at the large and
crowded house the patient was undressed, with
small show of gentleness, by several young women,
and placed at once in a crib, on straw, and fastened
to it by the feet, her hands being confined by iron
hand-locks, and a tight waistcoat put round the
trunk of the body and round her arms, the offices
of the nurses concluding for the time with the
administration of a dose of purgative salts. When
the patient, not yet forgetful of the decencies of
life, asked what she was to do if she wanted to get
out of bed, the nurses, hardened by their vocation,
merely answered her in the most vulgar terms.
Having in this miserable restraint become dirty,
which was inevitable, the patient was taken out of
bed, carried to the pump, and pumped upon with
cold water, and then, undried, taken back to her
crib, and fastened down again, but on fresh straw,
an attention not then in all cases considered necessary. All her remonstrances to the women about
her were laughed at. At this distant period she
still remembered her own expressions and theirs—

her appeals to them as women, her prayers for pity, and their too ready reply, which shut out hope— " You don't know what a madhouse is yet, but we will teach you." In the same room there were, she remembered, several maniacs, all in chains or restraints of some kind, singing, swearing, beating the walls. This scene, and her aggravated wretchedness, made her worse; and as she could not get up and move about, she could only sing or shout aloud, like the rest. For six weeks she was kept in that place of torment, and in those restraints; and, like most of the patients of those old asylums, the story of her restraints was written in broad indelible scars on her wrists, but in still worse characters on her memory. This patient remained for some time at Hanwell after relating these things to me, and was conducted safely through many severe paroxysms without the necessity of resorting to any restraints, for which her thanks were often expressed.

There were some patients in the asylum who had acquired so indifferent a character as never to be entrusted with perfect liberty of limbs. They were accused of frequently and suddenly striking or kicking those near them; or of pursuing the officers of the asylum and attempting to strangle them. Consequently, some of them had walked about for years with their hands fastened, and others had hobbled about the wards for as long a time with leathern leg-locks fastening their ankles together. With some misgivings, scarcely avoidable, as to the results, all these patients were set free ; the strikers for a time wore soft gloves—something like a boxing-glove—to make their sudden blows harmless ; and the rest were wholly trusted to. I do not recollect one of these cases in which any inconvenient result followed ; but I well remember some of them alluding to their happy liberation from their daily bondage years afterward.

In the large pauper asylums near London or any of our larger towns, the characters of the patients are more strongly marked, in general, than in the agricultural districts. They have been for the most part actively engaged in, and educated by, the multifarious accidents of a town life, and their faculties sharpened in the daily conflict of a crowd. Their passions have also been roused by perpetual excitements, and their vices have often spread widely under evil influences. The trouble occasioned by some patients of this kind is scarcely to be described. Of these we had many at Hanwell. As long as restraints were employed, several of them were rarely at complete liberty ; the attendants and patients equally dreaded them. But even in these patients, the effects of quiet treatment and of inexhaustible patience were generally seen at last: sometimes, however, after so long a period that all hope of their amendment had almost died away.

Among the older patients, in whose cases these characteristics had occasioned their being kept for years in restraints, the most melancholy examples were to be found of hopeless ferocity, upon which the altered state of the house produced little or no effect. It happened that some remarkable examples of the severest forms of mania were admitted on the female side of the asylum precisely when the gradual diminution of restraints was in progress. The subjects of some of these were women of middle age, who had been handsome, and who possessed considerable acuteness of intellect, ingenuity and activity, but whose lives had been a sort of troubled romance. Profligate, intemperate, violent, regardless of domestic ties, their children abandoned to all the evils of homeless poverty, themselves by degrees given up to utter recklessness—they had been the cause of ruin and shame to their families, and the history of their wild life had closed with madness. Others, and not a few, were the victims of the vices of those of a station superior to them, and left at length to struggle with difficulties and mortifications and remorse, beneath which reason gave way. In these patients all violent methods produced greater obstinacy, greater determination to give trouble, to do mischief, and to commit all kinds of outrages. It was not until such patients, in whatever mood of mind, found themselves treated, month after month, and even year after year, with invariable temper and patience, and nothing done to them that could be construed into punishment, that they became generally quiet, decorous in manners and language, attentive to their dress, disposed to useful activity, and able to preserve their good behaviour in the chapel. But these gratifying changes were in several instances strikingly exemplified.

Other cases there were, more pleasing as well as interesting, in which the educated faculties of the patients created facilities for remedial appliances of a mental kind, and where a gradual recovery revealed the various virtues of the human character, chastened by the many trials of humble life. The beautiful varieties of work executed by these patients in their convalescent state were often shown to admiring visitors, unprepared for such things in the wards of a lunatic asylum. All these circumstances give an animation to all parts of these large town institutions, of which the want is almost painfully perceived when those accustomed to such a lively throng of patients walk through the silent galleries of provincial asylums. Some of my descriptions, and even of my general remarks, may, I feel conscious, seem overstrained, because drawn from an institution where there is continual movement and variety; where the patients converse freely and much, and with great vivacity; where the manifestations of morbid mind are largely diversified, and where also the mental resources applicable to the alleviation of the patients are multiplied by these circumstances, with a corresponding variety of effect upon their lively intellects.

It happens that the greatest number of the illustrations I adduce are from the female side of the asylum, where, perhaps, the most striking instances occurred, and where, certainly, more attention was paid to the results. But cases of the same kind were not wanting on the male side, where restraints repeatedly resorted to, and hobbles worn for years, were taken off and consigned to the store-room, with every possible advantage to the patients. The greater strength of some of them had often filled some locality with alarm before they were secured, and they came to us bound up from head to foot with cords. They arrived at the asylum in a state of mixed fury and sullenness; sometimes, after a burst of violence, throwing themselves on the ground, refusing to speak or move, and not quite safe to approach. This violent state occasionally made it impracticable to bring them before the committee for inspection. But in a few days confidence seldom failed to be imparted even to these patients. They found that no bonds were put upon them; they heard themselves kindly addressed, and always in words without reproach; and observed that they were surrounded with

K

decencies and comforts. In such cases the mind, in many male patients, by degrees recovered its tone, and recovery was rapid and complete. And when taking leave of their kind officers and attendants in the asylum, they would now and then tell us that on admission they only fancied they had been sent to a new place of punishment and ill-treatment; and that they were surprised when they found themselves treated patiently and kindly; and that all at once they then began to feel as if they should get well.

In the first three months of my residence at Hanwell, I was often put out of countenance when walking with any visitors in the front grounds of the asylum, by finding myself hailed by name, and in a loud voice, from a window on the male side of the house, and reproached with cruelty and indifference to the speaker's situation; shut up, and handcuffed and leg-locked. I usually took an early opportunity of going into the man's room, and questioning him and the attendants of his ward respecting the reason of his being shut up, and in restraint. Finding that in almost every instance it arose from his having been passionate and threatening the attendants, and that he had on some occasions been strapped to his bed for days or weeks, with his hands enveloped in a leathern muff, and left to shout and rave until he was hoarse, I took various occasions of talking to him, both when

he was fastened and when he was at liberty; and
although generally finding that the attendants had
been as much in fault as the patient, I tried to
persuade him not to be so noisy, and especially not
to vociferate and abuse me for accidents which his
own irritability was the cause of. He would argue
against this; and often show that he had been
unjustly treated first, and then shut up for punishment; and he commonly concluded his argument
by saying that I should always find that if I tied
up a dog, the dog would howl. At length I forbade
the attendants to put him in restraints, under any
pretext, desiring them to send for me if the patient
was at any time particularly troublesome. Nearly
a year then elapsed without his becoming violent.
A paroxysm then came on, and he broke the door
of his room. Finding him after that outbreak disposed to talk quietly, it was stipulated that the door
of his room should not be locked, and his violence
did not return. In a few weeks afterward he was
well enough to attend the services in the chapel.
From that time there was scarcely ever a violent
scene with this man. He was very lively, very
friendly with myself, and lavish of titles and honours
on any friends who accompanied me through the
wards. He gradually became well enough to assist
the servants now and then in waiting at the officers'
tables. His case was not curable; and after a year
or two he died in the asylum. Very often, and at

last on his death-bed, this poor man would begin to allude to my having released him from almost habitual restraint; but he never could get on, so strong was the remembrance, and so acute his feeling on the subject: his voice invariably faltered and his eyes filled with tears. It was impossible not to derive additional determination to abolish all restraints for ever, when sitting by this poor declining man's side.

In the years that followed, instances were constantly occurring of patients arriving at the asylum in very unpromising states of bodily health, and in a very irritable state of mind, whose condition seemed to be more the product of protracted ill-treatment than of mere malady. Several of the male patients admitted were much emaciated, very dirty, and had extensive ulcerations on the back : sometimes the weakness of their lower limbs gave them the appearance of being paralysed. They were usually sullen, suspicious, and disposed to be violent. There was every reason to believe that both the bodily and mental condition had been produced or aggravated by straw beds, neglect, and restraints. Relieved from these disadvantages, their bodily health became gradually improved, and they became able to move about actively, and eventually got well. In one case of this kind the patient was a German musician; he was perfectly wild and incoherent, ran about the ward, hid his face, threw summersets, and was never at rest, and would scarcely take food. It was observed that when he wished to lie down he had recourse to singular positions in order to prevent the painful effects of pressure on his back. He had evidently been for some time fastened down in some asylum or workhouse. Being allowed perfect freedom of action at Hanwell, and having good food and porter, and exercise out of doors, the ulcerations healed, his strength improved; and, his naturally lively disposition returning, his skilful performances on the flute and the violin soon became a source of frequent gratification to the other patients, who much regretted his departure when he became too well to remain with us.

Patients are occasionally received at Hanwell whose mental derangement has thrown them out of very respectable stations into pauperism, and whose minds have been trained for pursuits or professions demanding ability. Early in 1844, a remarkable case of this kind occurred, in which the available resources of the patient had for some time secured for him the unhappy privilege of being treated in a private residence, under the care of two attendants. When his limited funds were exhausted, and his wife and children had become nearly penniless, a reluctant consent was obtained to his being sent to the county asylum, and, of course, as a pauper. He was about thirty

years of age, and prepossessing in his appearance;
but in his manner he was maniacal, and his
dangerous actions were only limited by his inability
to run about, in consequence of a lameness of
both legs, which it was feared arose from paralysis.
But it appeared that his two attendants, after
the daily visit of his physician, had been in the
habit of fastening him down in his bed; in which
state he had usually remained a great part of
every day, and all night, for several weeks; an
arrangement which left his attendants at liberty
to amuse themselves, or to sleep, regardless of
their charge. Being confined by no bonds at
Hanwell, although for a time he continued maniacal
and troublesome, and was irritated by finding himself in a crowd of patients whom he discerned
not to be of his own rank in life, his natural
amiability of disposition began to re-appear; his
confidence was gained; he became able to contemplate his position calmly; and at length resumed
his reading of works before familiar to him; and
patiently waiting until we thought him well enough
to go away, he cheerfully lent assistance for a
time in keeping the steward's books. His lameness
quite disappeared. We had afterward the satisfaction of learning that, after his discharge from
the asylum, he met the difficulties which confronted
him in the world with courage and patience, and
was soon actively and honourably employed. The

solitude of a cottage, and the idle negligence of attendants, and daily and nightly restraints, acting much longer on such a mind in illness, would in all probability have destroyed its power for ever.

These cases are not exceptional, or even selected as more particularly striking than many others. Instances of a like description abound in the Hanwell case-books; and the immediate improvement of the patients under the treatment pursued there, taken together with the state of the patients on admission, fully justified a belief that if the severe and negligent treatment to which the patients were almost uniformly subjected before coming to Hanwell had been prolonged, death would have been the result in many of the cases, and long retarded recovery in all the rest.

I might, indeed, enlarge this portion of my work to a great extent, and refer to very numerous cases of patients admitted to Hanwell, whose amendment began with the first kind care extended to them on admission, spoken of by themselves, when recovered, as the first kind care they had known in their distress. Some of these, having been described in my annual reports, made in successive years from 1839 to 1850, will be found mentioned in the extracts from those reports in Part IV. of this volume.

PART III.

THE NEW SYSTEM IN PRIVATE ASYLUMS.

THE principles which have been illustrated by examples drawn from a large county asylum, have been subsequently carried out, but with more difficulty, in several private establishments. They were, however, soonest carried into effect in the private asylums of which the proprietors were resolutely determined to overcome all obstacles, and to extend to richer patients the benefits already enjoyed by the pauper. The chief obstacles, indeed, were the want of a sufficient number of efficient attendants, and an indisposition to procure them. An excessive desire of gain had been, more than cruelty, the general cause of those gradually accumulating evils which had brought disgrace on many of the old institutions. The owners of lucrative private establishments were not content with moderate profits, but sought to make fortunes;

and any changes which interfered with these views were regarded with bitter hostility. Even to this day, there are private asylums in which the patients lead a life of wretched seclusion; and are subjected to indignities and severities which have long been unknown in public institutions. If we suppose a case in which the removal of a lady or a gentleman to a private asylum has become neces-sary, the difference between removal to a good and to a bad asylum is no less real than in the case of the poorest lunatic. The difference is even felt more keenly in consequence of the higher mental cultivation and more developed sensibility of the richer patient, who has in most cases a consciousness of mental failure or impairment, and an appreciation of the sacrifice of home, and of transference to a residence adapted to insane persons. These feelings make the interval between resolving on the removal and carrying it into effect full of danger and anxiety ; escape, or violence, or suicide, being peculiarly incidental to it. The patient, however, may yield to persuasion, or submit to force, and the removal takes place. The journey is often one of extreme excitement; the patient addresses the passers-by, or makes attempts to get out of the carriage. Fits of gloom and fits of passion occupy him by turns, and now and then his short suspicious questions reveal the apprehen-sions that prevail in his mind. When the journey, which seems to those who accompany him as if it would never end, is brought to a termination, his earnest but silent observation of all the objects near him, and of the house which they are approaching, is generally very remarkable, and still indicates the prevalence of suspicion and fear. For these feelings, indeed, the general aspect as well as character of the old private asylums afforded as much ground as the larger prisons for the destitute insane. Such houses were generally distinguishable from all the houses in the neighbourhood by their dismal appearance: their exterior was as gloomy as their interior was dirty. Heavy gates, a neglected shrubbery, windows heavily barred, doors clumsily locked, prepared the visitor for rooms which, although rooms of reception, had an air of cold discomfort and shabby finery; and whilst the friends of the patient were shown into them, the patient himself, ushered by men of repulsive aspect, disappeared into long passages, closed to the curiosity of those who brought him there in the hope that change of scene, and specific skill, and kindness, would promote his speedy recovery.

From that time, and commonly for a long period, the visits of all his friends were jealously interdicted; although the patient often grieved no less than they did at such absolute and prolonged denial of what might have been a consolation to

both. If the patient had previously been violent,
or had on any occasion acted in a manner to
excite a suspicion of a suicidal tendency, it was
not unusual to resort to restraint at once, and he
passed his first dreadful night in the asylum fast
bound in a strait-waistcoat. In the morning he
awoke to find himself in a strange apartment,
watched rather than waited upon by rude ungentle
keepers ; all the details of his dressing disregarded,
and his morning meal brought to him with little
care. An ill furnished, ill cleaned room, a half
darkened window, looking into a wretched yard,
and a scanty fire rendered less efficient for warmth
by a heavy fire-guard advancing far into the room,
were the characteristics of the apartment in which
he was to pass the day, either in solitude, or with
some other patients more or less afflicted than
himself. If he went out for exercise, it was into
a dolorous space of ground ; the grassplots and
borders of walks half trodden into clay, unadorned
by flowers, and disfigured rather than ornamented
by torn and withering shrubs and trees. The
hour of dinner brought no comfortable meal ; and
no social or rational conversation, and no amusements of any kind, diversified the evening. Beyond
the boundaries of the lofty walls no exercise was
allowed ; and within them there was no variety
and no companionship, nor any thing calculated
to cheer the mind or soothe the feelings ; so that

by degrees even the hope of change and liberation became faint, and almost died away. Such, I know from observation made when the access of visitors to such establishments was difficult, and my own visits were only permitted because an official appointment qualified me to demand it, was the general condition of insane persons in the old asylums; in which the doctrine of non-restraint was years afterward received with derision and defiance, and made the groundwork of every kind of misrepresentation ; and into which the full principle of non-restraint can scarcely yet be said to have found a willing admission.

Incidental to my position at Hanwell has been, in the course of years, the receipt of communications from several persons, in various parts of the kingdom, descriptive of their sufferings in private asylums; sufferings for which there seemed to be no redress. In one memorable instance, the wife of a man of great wealth, concerning whom I had been consulted when she was affected with recent puerperal insanity, was removed, without my advice or knowledge, to a provincial asylum of considerable pretensions, and admitted there on expensive terms. Being suddenly removed from a luxurious home, and from her children and relatives and a most indulgent husband, she was received with a great show of interest : but it being mentioned that her malady had sometimes shown itself in self-reproach, dejection,. and an apparent disregard of life, this poor lady, who was highly accomplished and sensitive, and remarkable for her tender and compassionate character, was taken from the drawing-room on the very evening of her arrival, fastened up in a strait-waistcoat for the night, and left alone. In a strange place, and, for the first time in her life, entirely surrounded by strange people, her sufferings may be imagined. Such was the first step, in such an establishment, to allay mental suffering. Its effects were described to me by herself after her convalescence ; and among many affecting expressions she said, " The tears of despair flowed fast from my eyes, and I could not even raise my hands to wipe them away." The painful impressions made on the mind of this lady will never be quite effaced. In the midst of the domestic duties to which she has long returned, and of benevolent exertions to which she devotes much time, recollections of the past still often sadden and affright her. Her letters to myself on the subject of her treatment in the asylum, on the harshness of the attendants, the prevalence of restraints, the consequent uncleanliness and wretchedness of the patients, and on the absence of all alleviating appliances, contain instructive lessons, less needful now than when penned but a few years ago ; but which are still unlearned in many places where they would be useful.

In this case, the convalescence of the patient, which she has often spoken of as awakening her to the character of her dismal room, &c., was not made known to her husband; and he was still denied, after a long and anxious journey, the consolation of seeing her. She herself had seen him arrive, and, after indulging in the hope of an interview, had to suffer all the agony of disappointment. The husband, almost broken-hearted, came straightway to Hanwell, to seek my advice; which was that he should immediately remove his wife to the residence of a medical friend near London. As soon as his intention to do so was communicated to the proprietor of the asylum, a letter was despatched assuring him that his wife was well, and that the proprietor had been about to write to that effect. The patient was at once removed; and, although not quite well, was convalescent, and soon afterward recovered entirely.

If such was the mode of treatment adopted in cases of patients of the richer class, and in which no violence existed, it may readily be supposed that the treatment of more troublesome cases, for which more limited payments were also made, was proportionably coarse and severe. In letters written by patients of this description after recovery, are to be found details which would appear incredible if they had not, on more than one occasion, been the subject of judicial investigation,

and proved to be true.   Fetters and chains,
moppings at the morning toilet, irregular meals,
want of exercise, the infliction of abusive words,
contemptuous names, blows with the fist, or with
straps, or with keys, formed almost a daily part of
the unprotected daily life of many wretched beings,
previously accustomed to comfort, and decency,
and kindness, and reasonable enough to feel the
bitterness of being debarred from all.   When they
became paralysed, and in some degree helpless,
they were consigned to coercion-chairs, the great
substitute for all care and attention : and in them
they sate, day after day, for years ; rendered for a
time more irritable, but at length falling into
imbecility, and èxposed to all the miseries consequent on systematic neglect.

Among the happy changes effected since a good
example was first set in the Friends' Retreat at
York, are now to be found private houses for those
afflicted in mind where all is different, and where
everything is calculated to assuage the fear of a
newly arrived patient, to win confidence, and to
tranquillize and restore the mind.   The outward
appearance of such houses is indicative of comfort :
highly cultivated grounds and gardens surround
them, and nothing is suggestive of a place of
confinement.   The patient is received as a visitor,
proper refreshment is placed before him, friendly
words are addressed to him, and he retires at night

to a bed-room where cleanliness and all arrangements fitting to his station in life reconcile him to
being its occupant. If his case requires that an
attendant should be near him in the night, or even
in the same room with him, it is represented to
him that this is done for his own safety or for his
comfort in a strange house. In the morning he is
persuaded to get up, without threats and rough
words, and his dressing is attended to as carefully
as if he were in his own house. On coming down
stairs he finds a cheerful breakfast prepared for
him, either with a few other patients, or with one
of the proprietors or officers of the establishment.
He can read the morning paper, or walk out in the
grounds, or look over the new books from the
library, or adjourn to the billiard-room, or join one
of the walking parties, or carriage parties. On
returning, he is allowed, within limits of prudence,
and of rules necessary for the preservation of
health, to choose what luncheon he will take—a
small privilege, but productive of a feeling of liberty
not to be undervalued. The remainder of the
morning is passed much according to his own
inclination. The visits of friends to himself or the
other patients, or to the proprietors, and from
conversation with whom he is not debarred, diversi-
fies much of the time, and serves to introduce new
ideas without any formality of device ; and at
dinner time he sits down with the proprietor,

the resident physician, and perhaps a lady acting as matron, and with several of the patients who are gentlemen of his own station, and whose neatness of dress reminds him of the propriety of his making some alteration in his own before that meal. A table well appointed, an excellent and varied dinner, wine in moderation, a dessert, and agreeable conversation, make him almost unmindful of being the inmate of an asylum; and in the evening, a party in the drawing-room, and music, and chess, and backgammon, and cards, make the hours pass agreeably until it is time to retire.

If the patient is even in the acute stage of disorder, these arrangements prevail with modifications adapted to his state, and contribute to tranquillise him. Before the step of removal was taken, his life, for weeks, has usually been a distempered dream. He has talked and walked night and day; taken stimulants to relieve his exhaustion; he has been haunted by suspicions; pursued by imaginary voices; everything that he has heard, and everything that he has read, has seemed to be especially addressed to him; advertisements have been aimed at him, sermons directed against him, and popular authors have had him in their view. His food has been poisoned, his limbs have been magnetised, and signs and portents have appeared to him in the sky. His whole conduct has, consequently, been irregular and extravagant.

L

And all this hurricane subsides when his friends at length make up their minds to remove him, if, happily, he is taken to a good asylum.

More than once I have seen men of station and accomplishments in whom a gradual failure of mental power had previously caused considerable loss or wasting of their property ; and whom exalted delusions have led into the wildest extravagance. Fancying themselves persons of extraordinary importance, they had nearly worn themselves out in walking with restless and futile purposes to the public offices and palaces, sallying forth every morning full of great thoughts, and returning at night, without their money, or their rings, or their watches, having taken no food, and yet, although exhausted, still full of hope that the deficiencies of that day would be amply supplied on the morrow. When, at length, such persons have become sheltered in a good asylum, the delusive hopes have gently faded away, and left the mind calm ; the restless wanderings have given place to regular and health-ful exercise ; careful diet and regular hours have improved the physical health, and the patients have become stout and contented ; remaining incurable, and gradually advancing towards death, but enjoying rest and peace.

In private asylums for ladies, the same rules now obtain, and the same effects follow, modified only by obvious circumstances. All the resources of

female work and female accomplishments are called
into operation : including a greater variety of in-
door occupations ; and, if possible, a more scrupulously constant attention to dress, appearance,
manners, and language ; and to whatever, in
furniture, in amusement, or in regulated intercourse
with society, or with visitors, can afford variety
and pleasant excitement, maintained within harmless, and, therefore, within salutary, bounds.
Although the forms of their malady may be
various, and the symptoms at times distressing,
the greater number of lady-patients preserve a
recollection of music ; many are ingenious in needle-
work ; and others possess skill and acuteness in
games and recreations suitable to the sex : and
these acquirements, judiciously called into exercise,
subserve strongly to the alleviation of their mental
disorder, if not directly to recovery.   These may
appear not very important matters of detail ; but
the daily life of most men, and of most women, is
made up of small details, and, when important
occupations are withdrawn, the details become
limited to such as have been enumerated, and
which, in the aggregate, are of incomparable value
to the greater number of patients in private
asylums ; to women, severed from home associations
and domestic duties, and to men debarred from the
performance of all daily and customary occupations,
and from all habitual relaxations—from their club,

their ordinary rides and drives, the visits of their neighbours, and the society of their families. It is by the operation of such influences, and by the general and indirect effect of the new habits of life induced in a good asylum, and substituted for the perverted habits of disordered minds—it is by the impressions there made, and also by the impressions from thence excluded, that the great majority of patients are more benefited than by the direct effect of medicines. Of few medicines can it yet be confidently asserted that they are strikingly useful in the generality of the cases of insanity ; whilst few can be conveniently administered in those forms of the disease in which medicinal aid seems most urgently to be required, and would probably be most efficacious, if the administration of medicine were practicable. Those of which the direct efficacy is the most established are almost limited in their application to cases of melancholia. The great medicine, therefore, in numerous cases, is the separation of the patient from all the circumstances which surrounded him when he became insane, and placing him in the centre of new and salutary influences.

The state of the mind of the insane often makes them, indeed, more satisfied with the new life they lead in the asylum than with the old life they led at home, for which a morbid restlessness had long unfitted them ; and they enjoy the companionship

and occupations of their new abode so completely
as to prevent their regretting the absence of old
friends, and the entire suspension of all their
ordinary employments and pursuits. Certain
harassing trains of thought appear to be interrupted by the change, with relief to the distressed
mind; whilst numerous unsalutary associations are
put an end to by the presence of new scenes and
new people.

As respects lady-patients, so long as they remain
at home, all domestic influences usually cease to
benefit them ; they live in an insane reverie.
Religious ecstacy, or deep despondency, occupies
them : voices from heaven have enjoined abstinence
from food, or the abandonment of all their
domestic duties; sometimes they have been declared,
as they believe, to be the bride of Christ, and
counselled to suicide as a means of joining their
heavenly bridegroom. From all their relatives
they have been quite estranged ; all their conduct
has been fierce and unnatural; life itself, perhaps,
in constant jeopardy. In the meantime, the
habitation of the family has been full of anxiety
or terror. The remotest parts of it have been
rendered awful by the presence of a deranged
creature under the same roof : her voice ; her
sudden and violent efforts to destroy things or
persons ; her vehement rushings to fire and
window; her very tread and stamp in her dark and

disordered and remote chamber, have seemed to penetrate the whole house; and, assailed by her wild energy, the very walls and roof have appeared unsafe, and capable of partial demolition. To all these sources of alarm, removal to a good asylum puts an immediate end. The malady remains, but the terror is gone; and whilst by the patient's being removed to an asylum, the friends are thus relieved from disturbance and dread, the situation of the patient herself undergoes no less happy a change. The strait-waistcoat, and all the ingenious bonds resorted to by frightened servants and nurses at home, are at once removed; and if she continues excited and violent she is placed in a secure room, not darkened, but having the fire - place and windows protected; and presenting no very ready means of offensive measures being successful. An interval is allowed for the supervention of calmness, or of some approach to it. The case is medically examined; and all that course of mingled kindness and caution is commenced and persevered in of which the many details have been already described. The wider range of moral causes affecting educated persons receives due attention; and attempts to soothe the mind are made without rashness, and only as favourable times occur for such attempts. All the conversation addressed to them is discreet. The physical condition is diligently inquired into; and functions manifestly disordered are rectified

by appropriate remedies.   The real cause of the
malady is sought for either in these bodily
derangements, or in the previous habits of the
patient, or in circumstances which may have
suddenly or slowly disturbed the brain.   The
tendency of long-continued irritation to produce
structural change is remembered ; and the frail
tenure of life in recent and violent mania is not
forgotten.   As immediate consequences, all excitement of mind, and all bodily irritation, all foolish
indulgence, and all exciting topics of discussion,
are carefully avoided.   To tranquillise and to cure,
and not merely to subdue, being the object, nothing
in the treatment is at variance with the great
system of non-restraint prevailing throughout the
establishment.

A fatal result has, I am convinced, been occasioned, not unfrequently, in recent maniacal cases,
merely by violent coercion, and its usual accom-
paniment of neglects.   Two young ladies, sisters,
became a few years ago, by some accident, or some
strange sympathy, insane at the same period of
time, in their mother's house.   They were kept at
home, two nurses being engaged to attend to them
in an out-of-the-way bedroom containing two beds.
The nurses discovered that one of the easiest ways
of lightening their own labours, was to tie each
of these young ladies to the bed-posts of their
respective beds ; and the poor maniacal girls

exerted their morbid energy in dragging the bedsteads about after them. In less than a month, the weakest of the two sunk and died. The survivor, reduced almost to a shadow, was then removed to a good asylum, where the only restraint was kindness. For a few days she was furious; and then her joy at finding herself still left at liberty found expression in peals of wild laughter; and then, in succession, the excitement subsided, convalescence was gradually established, life was preserved, and health of body and mind restored. It was from this lady's own lips, after recovery, that I heard the story of her first sufferings, and of that sad companionship which death had ended: of much of which, even when most excited, she seemed to have been conscious.

The difficulties to be met in many cases increase in proportion to the previous cultivation of the patient's mind, or the peculiar studies which have been pursued, and the wider range of her imagination. Accomplished women, naturally religious, and who have perplexed themselves by controversial theological reading, and thoughts beyond the reaches of their souls, are prone to imagine their condition and prospects hopeless here and hereafter. They sometimes imagine that for their individual sins the government of the world has been given up to an evil spirit; the solar heat is increased; blazing writings are legible in the air; and they are themselves to be destroyed by fire from heaven. These and other terrible thoughts will disappear for a time, and re-appear suddenly and dangerously, generally accompanied with an impulse to destroy life; so that suicide is attempted in many ingenious ways, demanding long and incessant care. But life has again and again been preserved by such care, without any resort to restraints; and recovery has at length followed when the patients have been for some time removed from home influences, and placed in an asylum. Extraordinary amendment sometimes takes place immediately after removal. Gentlemen of education and refinement, who have refused to be dressed, or washed, or shaved for long periods together, and ladies for whom not any service of the toilet could be performed without violent resistance—who have refused to be dressed or undressed, or to walk out—have, in cases under my own observation, even after disorderly years of this kind of life, submitted, immediately after their arrival at a comfortable asylum, to take a warm bath, and then to be properly dressed in all respects; and no subsequent contention of any importance has afterward arisen out of the daily care taken to keep them clean in person and neat in dress, and regular as to habits of food and exercise and rest. Others who have kept their families in a perpetual state of disturbance for a length of time, and have persisted in being up all night and in bed all the day, with arbitrary and most inconvenient hours for meals, or for walking out, have, under the altered circumstances attendant on removal to a good asylum, conformed at once to the hours and customs of the house. Consequent on these changes, an infinite number of small improvements take place. Slovenly or disgusting habits in the manner of taking food, and negligence as to all matters of cleanliness, give way to orderly practices, and even to scrupulous neatness. Customary occupations long interrupted, exercise long neglected, social conversation long shunned or almost forgotten for want of opportunities, and a lively interest in persons and things around them, gradually form a part of their daily asylum life. Patients transferred from asylums conducted on the old plan to the improved asylums of this time, present the most striking examples of the results of opposite modes of treatment. A man of rank comes in, ragged, and dirty, and unshaven, and with the pallor of a dungeon upon him; wild in aspect, and as if crazed beyond recovery. He has passed months in a lonely apartment, looking out on a dead wall; generally fastened in a chair. He has the appearance of a mad beggar; and all decent habitudes seem to have been forgotten. Liberty to walk at all hours of the cheerful day in gardens or fields, and care and attention, metamorphose him into the well dressed and well bred gentleman he used to be ; he discontinues various habits and antics, the growth of solitude and vacuity of mind and heart; and the colour of health is equally restored to his complexion and to his thoughts.   In time, the tranquil days and nights, the regularity of hours of exercise and meals, good diet, cheerful social intercourse, and hopeful words often heard, together with the administration of baths, and all the medical and therapeutic means practicable as well as obviously necessary in some cases, produce a permanent impression on the whole frame of body and mind. The general health, usually much interrupted in maniacal and melancholic cases, is greatly improved, or quite re-established ; the expression of the patient's countenance, so singularly altered by mental disorder, becomes natural ; the whole appearance of the patient improves ; the circulation becomes tranquillised ; the functions of the nervous system become normally performed ; and delusions vanish, and the judgment is re-established, and the patient is cured.   If a cure is in certain cases impossible, at least the worst features of the malady disappear.   Nothing occurring, from day to day, to exasperate the patient; no unkind thing being ever done ; no unkind expression ever addressed to him; no ungentle emotion ever roused ; the patient's hours and days glide on in peace and content; his nights become habitually tranquil;

and his calmer state is shown in his mode of dressing himself, and of walking, and of eating, and of talking, and in the altered expression of his face, and in short, in all that he says or does.

Effects of this kind, so generally and remarkably exhibited in a good asylum, irresistibly suggest the idea that if all people were as careful not to provoke their fellow-creatures to wrath as the officers of such asylums are; were as indulgent to faults, and as accustomed to encourage and aid all attempts at self-control and improvement; and if, which cannot be, the sane were as much secured, in the liberty of the world, as the insane are in their retreat from it, from want and knawing care, the world without the walls of such places would far more abound in happiness, and far less in the causes by which so many distracted minds are driven within them for shelter and relief of a distempered brain, become so in the distempered life in which their irremediable hurt has been incurred. When the day arrives in which mankind, alarmed by the spreading of insanity, begin to pay some rational attention to its causes, although some of those causes will be found inseparable from our imperfect state, many may be discovered to be the mere product of arrangements modifying human life and character from the earliest years ; concurred in, without reflection, by one generation after another, but as capable of removal as are the

various influences so long permitted to prevail with
pernicious effects on the physical health of communities, and only now beginning to receive full
and general attention.   Very little consideration is
required to show that in the management of children
of tender years, many customs prevail which directly
tend to irritate and spoil the growing brain.   The
system of mental and physical training generally
adopted for children and youth of either sex, and
their general treatment, are so far from being
adapted to secure a sound mind in a sound body
as to be little better than a satire on the common
sense of mankind.   From the very beginning,
nothing is so conspicuous as a steady disregard of
physiological principles.   In cases in which con-
genital defect is obvious, and imbecility in its
various afflicting forms is clearly recognised, institutions of modern date are happily open for relief,
and for systematic education.   In these schools,
all of modern institution, the character of each
pupil receives serious preliminary inquiry : qualities
which appear naturally defective are not forced;
faculties congenitally feeble are, if possible, strengthened, but never stimulated to diseased exertion;
the moral qualities claim especial consideration;
what is faulty and wrong is soon associated with a
certain shame and sorrow; what is good and
praiseworthy receives generous encouragement.
Whilst the intellect is trained, the affections are

tenderly cultivated. At the same time it is not forgotten that the imperfect mind is enclosed in an imperfect body; and all the physical aids that science has dictated, and ingenuity has devised, are brought to bear, as far as practicable, on each case. The very imperfection of these little beings secures for them an education more comprehensive than that which is considered worthy of attention as regards children of average capacity.

But there are juvenile victims not a few, wayward and eccentric, with faculties unequally developed, but yet not so marked with malady as to be preserved from ordinary modes of education, and even from undertaking some of the preliminary duties of life ; in which, soon failing, they cease to be regarded ; are thrown down in a crowd where they are unfitted to compete ; trampled on, and put aside. The physician whose business occupies him with the infirmities of mind, then, perhaps, sees even these unsuccessful beings brought, in ruinous state, to places in which, as creatures grievously stricken, they are at last privileged to find refuge. But there are others still labouring in the walks of life, not so obviously afflicted as to be withdrawn from exertions in which they never succeed, and scenes in which their lot can only be to suffer. For many of these it would have been a happy circumstance if they had been educated in institutions where alone the common principles of physiology

are applied to the development of the understanding
and the control of the feelings.   Many a wayward
temper, inherited from half insane ancestors, might
thus be soothed and regulated, and many young
persons spared many years of wretchedness, of
useless efforts, of errors and vices which reflect
pain and grief on those to whom, defective as
they are become, and faulty, they still remain dear,
if their early years could be passed in institutions
adapted to their feeble intellect and violent passions.
Attempts to amend these inherited or acquired
faults by severities are never successful.   Unlimited
indulgence is equally fatal.   Ordinary education,
pursued with no higher views than the acquisition
of fortune or station, has no salutary result.   The
time may come in which it may be found that there
are duties in this high department for officers of
health, who have studied the laws of body and
mind, and who will be listened to when they point
out the various follies to which the temper, and
the feelings, and the understanding of successive
generations, in this civilized, enlightened, and
religious country (for so we deem it), are sacrificed;
and why, when the most precious fruits of the
mind should appear, they are so often overlaid
by selfishness, and perish or wither in the air of
unwholesome metaphysics, medicine, and religion,
wafted from phantom-lands, and spread over
societies as a wide epidemic.   As it is, in each

revolving year we see that no mental speculation seems too hazardous, no magical trick and fancied influence too unreal, no medical doctrine too absurd, no prophesy of distorted faith and limited reasoning power too visionary to be trusted and pursued, in the place of fact, and truth, and "divine philosophy." The gates of asylums now open to receive many who have travelled to madness by the paths through which these fleeting fictions of the fancy have led them, and who have at length but embraced some unsubstantial cloud instead of heavenly beauty.

The time must come when man's reason will manifest itself more strongly in exercising the means of preserving his highest privileges; triumphing over errors of moral and physical education now so generally unfavourable to his nature, and often only recognised when they have overthrown the mind. All who have peculiar opportunities of ascertaining the mental habits of insane persons of the educated classes well know that, with some exceptions, their previous studies and pursuits appear to have been superficial and desultory, and often frivolous: the condition of the female mind, especially of the minds of those who are to be the mothers of another generation, is, even in the highest classes, too often more deplorable still. Not only is it most rare to find them familiar with the best authors of their own country, but most common to find that they have

never read a really good author either in their
own or in any other language, and that the few
accomplishments possessed by them have been
taught for display in society, and not for solace
in quieter hours. All this has been said before,
and often, and in vain. But there is a frequent
perversion of intellectual exercise more fatal than
its omission, and which fills asylums with lady
patients, terrified by metaphysical translations, and
bewildered by religious romances, and who have
lost all custom of healthful exertion of body or
mind, all love of natural objects, all interest in
things most largely influencing the happiness of
mankind. All the higher pleasures of human
beings have always been unknown to these patients.
Minds so feeble, or so spoiled, are unfit for the
ordinary emergencies of a chequered life. Every
stronger shock quite discomposes them. These
evils have generally taken deep root before the
patient's manifest want of reasonable control induces
a resort to an asylum; but a large portion of the
moral treatment resorted to in asylums consists in
the discouragement of the evil habits of mind into
which such frivolous and unhappy beings have
fallen. Exercise in the open air; customary and
general activity; regular hours; a moderate attention to music and other accomplishments instead
of an extravagant devotion of time to such excitements; protection from fanatical exhortations; and

M

the substitution of sensible books for the worthless
tracts and volumes with which their well-meaning
friends have generally loaded their boxes, and
which are thenceforth locked up as so much mental
poison, contribute largely to the patient's advance
towards rationality. The same kind of care might
in many cases have preserved the mind from
derangement; but the attention of parents and
teachers is seldom directed to the important object
of the prevention of insanity.

It is surprising and painful to observe how little
interest is really taken in education as a means to
this great end; although several able writers have,
during late years, published useful works connected
with physical as well as moral training. To some
of these all parents may have their attention
usefully directed; but more especially those whose
children manifest such intellectual or moral pecu-
liarities, combined with so peculiar a development
of the head, as evidently demand more than usual
consideration, and are calculated to create great
anxiety. Among the best may be mentioned the
late Dr. Andrew Combe's " Principles of Physiology
applied to the Preservation of Health and to the
Improvement of Physical and Mental Education,"
published in 1835; Dr. Southwood Smith's " Philosophy of Health," published in the same year;
Mr. Charles Bray's work on " The Education of
the Feelings;" and a small volume published by

Pickering, on "Man's Power over Himself to Prevent or Control Insanity," written by the Rev. John Barlow.   From these works may be gathered many directions for the regulation of the life of children, conformable in principle and in object to the character of the non-restraint system applied to older and more decidedly disordered minds.   By these they may be to a great extent instructed how to avert evils which, increasing and becoming established, are found most difficult to cure.

From the peculiar life led in asylums—all circumstances being excluded which ordinarily prove exciting to morbid minds—it usually results that the same man who, when at home, not only neglected his affairs, but wore out his strength in foolish exertions; wandering over the town or the country, and often returning ragged and destitute; or who was full of restless schemes, purchasing what was not wanted, and gradually ruining himself, becomes, almost from the moment of his reception into a comfortable asylum, quite tranquil and contented, and improves, not only in appearance, but in his mental state.   More violent patients, who have kept a whole neighbourhood in alarm, or have threatened injury to individuals by whom they imagined themselves wronged, become, in a good asylum, like men delivered at once from the fiercer passions and all the turbulent feelings that agitate the human heart; or if not always at once, generally to a considerable extent in the course of time. Many are conscious of the relief; and thus we find patients living in asylums by choice, or after occasional excursions into the outside world, returning as from a sea of troubles to a quiet haven. We meet with numerous instances in which those recovered come afterward to visit the asylum to which they were taken in the outbreak of their disorder, and where they remained till their affliction had subsided. The medical and other officers who attended to them, the attendants who watched them day and night, the children of the proprietors or physician, and even the servants, are inquired for in these visits, and recognised with various degrees of affection and gratitude. These are indications, not to be mistaken, of the mitigation they experienced there of mental sufferings scarcely appreciable by those to whom the disturbance of reason has never been known.

In a good asylum, then, everything acts favourably on the mind of the patient; a result impossible, in many cases, to be attained in the patient's home, and scarcely ever arrived at in an isolated residence. Everything is arranged to promote health of the body, and to maintain a peaceful mental state; so that as the bodily condition becomes composed and healthy, nothing counteracts its favourable action on the feelings and the understanding. The precise condition of the brain in different patients is, it

has been acknowledged, as little known as the mode
and nature of its actions in health.   The manner
in which its functions are interrupted or disordered
in insanity lies in a region beyond the reach of
man's senses, and seems scarcely a legitimate object
for strictly philosophical imagination, unaided by
any means of appreciating it, and leading merely
to "wandering thoughts and notions vain."   But
the connection of these actions with material organs,
and their evident sympathy with the body in health
and in disease, impart certain resources to the
physician; who, if he can only act directly on
the mind within narrow limits, finds that he can
extensively and powerfully influence it by sedulous
attention to the state of the temple in which, in
this condition of existence, it is enshrined.

There are, doubtless, exceptional and painful
cases in which the disorder is too general and
irremediable to admit even of much amelioration.
Severe and troublesome forms of malady are met
with in private as well as in public asylums in
which the mere appliances of social life are either
insufficient or inapplicable, and care and medicine
are alike, to a great extent, powerless.   There may
be maniacal violence, or profound melancholia, in a
considerable proportion of cases, combined even
with suicidal tendencies.   Such cases are treated
on the general principles already spoken of as
practised in public institutions; the treatment not

being left to uninstructed attendants, but carefully regulated by the physician and by efficient assistants. The destructive activity of the patient is guarded against, or his own safety secured against his own impulses, by the arrangements adopted in the rooms inhabited by those who are temporarily violent, and by constant superintendence. The transient duration of such states, in almost all cases, is always kept in view; and nothing is done to leave impressions on the patient's mind painful and unfavourable to subsequent recovery. Darkness and bonds are, even in these difficult cases, never applied; hasty and reproachful words are forbidden; punishment is a word unknown; and, as far as can be done in intervals of calmness, the patient is the object of soothing attentions; whilst, during the worst paroxysms of his disorder, he is never abandoned and left to his wretchedness.

It seems extraordinary that a most acute cerebral disorder may continue even for many months, and still end in recovery. In all that troubled time, there may have been no rest and no rationality; but perpetual movement and noise, or with, at the most, a few occasional hours of repose: yet the patient will recover, and sometimes recovers suddenly; and after all the involuntary actions of this prolonged excitement sometimes no fatigue ensues. Usually, however, recovery is prefaced by intervals of sensibility and recollection; by tears and depression; and at length the patient is observed to be altogether reasonable. Still, in these cases, neglect may wholly alter the event. Depression, also, may ensue, requiring undiminished vigilance; and this condition is most to be apprehended in persons of cultivated intellect; who more acutely feel the nature of their temporary loss of mental power, and dread the possibility of a return of so heavy an affliction. The depression is usually temporary; but there are sensitive individuals who live in fear of impending insanity ever afterward: a fear rendered less intolerable, however, than when insanity consigned them to the old places of reception, and a recurrence of illness menaced them with utter seclusion from the cheerful world.

In all asylums there are many patients whom no art can cure : yet the continual action of a system strictly humane modifies the character of such patients, with the result of making them useful even to the curable. The extravagances, the violent displays of eccentricity and passion, and all the painful consequences of mad conduct in ordinary society, are suppressed. General calmness and docility are gradually established; and their life is so regulated as to ensure them a share of comfort, and even of happiness, which is forfeited whenever the too impatient friends, who observe this restored capability of tranquil life, act on the delusive conviction that it will continue when the patient is unwisely set at large. Each experiment of this kind shows that the gentle superintendence of the asylum, present to the consciousness of the patient, effective, yet not oppressive, keep all the machinery of his mind in regular action. This gentle pressure removed, all flies into disorder; to the dismay of the friends, and seldom without detriment to the unfortunate patient himself.

There are still other patients, in private as well as public asylums, who are deprived, by the nature or by the stage of their mental affliction, of the higher advantages even of the best ordered treatment. Some of these lapse into mere imbecility, and in others paralysis ensues on mental excitement, and renders them powerless, and wholly dependent on the pure kindness of those about them. For these, in the old days, a desolate apartment, a sloping stone floor, a stable-gutter, and coercion-chairs, were the common substitutes for care and superintendence. The more humane system of the present time extends especial attention to these cases, and repudiates the dreadful idea that because the patients are helpless they are insensible; and that a chair from which they cannot wander, and from which they cannot fall, with accompaniments of cold and dirt and famine, and a bed of straw in which they can be fastened at night, are all the requirements of their unhappy condition. The infirmaries of our pauper asylums in all the counties of England, or in nearly all, have now for many years shown that on no class of insane patients has humanity been more actively exerted than on these. The same care has since been happily introduced into all good private institutions. Comfortable chairs, safe, but without the apparatus of chairs of coercion; great care as to preserving cleanliness; systematic attention to food, dress, and to the comfort of the patient's bed, cause these most helpless of all the inmates of an asylum to be of all perhaps the most comfortable and cheerful. As long as they can move about, their placid and satisfied state, or their childlike vivacity, are remarkable. The more intellectual of them still project great undertakings; or fancy themselves engaged in important literary compositions; or please themselves with the hope of large advancement. Toward those around them they exercise an imaginary and most generous patronage; offering them wealth, or conferring honours and rank upon them. They are themselves treated as tenderly as children, and thus continue for the most part harmless; but they are easily irritated, and any harshness shown to them reproduces painful exhibitions of weakness and anger, common in the old days, when they were generally all submitted to some form or other of coercion. When, later still, they can scarcely exercise voluntary movements, friendly and protecting arms are extended to aid their steps. When they can walk no longer, every resource of comfortable rest is provided for them ; including that great boon to the afflicted, the water-bed of Dr. Arnott ; on which they sometimes lie for many months before death, free from abrasions or suffering, their malady mercifully softened even to the close of life.

In a small private asylum, no less than in a larger institution for insane persons, everything must be arranged with a constant regard to the inmates for whom it is intended. It must be remembered that asylums are filled with those in whom either reverses, or violent mental emotions, or ill regulated passions, or domestic troubles, or long-continued trials and disappointments, or the poverty of successive generations resulting in deteriorated nervous structure and development, have produced disorder in the action of the human brain. Morbid excitement, or a suspension of nervous energy and consequent depression, with various impairments of thought, feeling, and action, have supervened in some degree or other ; and exist in every case that is admitted. Therefore, as in an hospital for the cure of bodily maladies everything is carefully arranged to restore and to secure bodily health—and the diet, the air, the temperature, and all other circumstances are studiously regulated to this end—so, in a lunatic

asylum, there should be no source of violent
emotion or passion, nor of disappointment or
sorrow ; no rudeness, no deception, no strife, no
want, and no excess. Thus all the ordinary causes
of agitation being excluded, the natural tendency
to restore the balance of health is exercised in the
brain and nerves without interruption; and the
timely and judicious administration of remedies is
found successful; and, where no structural change
has yet taken place incapable of removal, the
patient is calmed, or consoled, and recovers the
blessing of reason: whilst in cases wherein organic
and irremoveable mischief already exists, or painful
complications of disease and infirmity have supervened, no alleviation is wanting by which suffering
and irritation can be diminished, and tranquillity
of mind preserved ; so that, although troubled
with occasional interruptions, and temporary
ruffling, the current of the patient's life flows on
smoothly, not without many comforting gleams of
brightness.

By a combination of all the means now enumerated, judiciously combined, and modified,so as to
meet the countless shades of mental malady,
private and public asylums for the insane have
become no longer places over which the veil of
oblivion is thrown by those who consign their
afflicted relatives to them ; but real places of

refuge; homes of peace, and of recovery from all
the mental distractions incidental to mankind.   Of
those who enter them, few or none are utterly
devoid of understanding or affection.   Some share
of 'both commonly remains ; and to these unex-
tinguished remains are applied all the agencies
that can kindle their energy anew, and restore
their power.   Society is thus at first and at once
protected from the consequences that might result
from the dangerous irregularities of human beings
whose guiding reason is impaired ; and then the
frame of mind and body is carefully inspected,
with a view to restoring in each case, as far as may
be possible, the active and regular exercise of the
intellect, and the healthful flow of the affections,
and the consequent restraint of the propensities
within safe and reasonable bounds, consistent with
the restoration of liberty.   But all this constitutes
a task demanding the devotion of the physician's
whole heart to it.   He must have a constant sense
of what each hour of the day requires from him,
and be accurately, even minutely, acquainted with
what is hourly taking place in all parts of the
establishment.   No action, no expression, no voice,
no sound in the whole building, however large,
must be at variance with that even, tranquil,
calming system which is adapted to allay, or
certainly not to increase, the troubles of the brain.
Everywhere it must be felt that his *mind*, at least,

is present : he must superintend, and mingle with, and partake of, all that constitutes the daily life of his patients : so that every arrangement may be part of an harmonious system of which he is the soul ; and every patient, according to the extent of his faculties, may still know that in all his afflictions and troubles, the physician is his sure and constant friend.

Such, then, is the non-restraint system ; by which it is found to be no less practicable, and safe, and advantageous, to control, and govern, and in many cases to contribute to the cure, and in all to the improvement of the insane, in private than in public asylums : a system which meets all the difficulties arising out of the condition of the most highly endowed creature in the universe when deprived of guiding reason, and when, in proportion to his higher faculties and gifts, he has fallen from being either in reason noble, or in faculty infinite, to a condition in which he is merely the most mischievous, and dangerous, and miserable of animals. In the illustrative cases already given, the applicability of this system, which excludes all forms of mechanical coercion, has, I think, been shown in relation to every form of mental imbecility, derangement, depression, and decay. The general results are open to all observation in all our larger asylums ; — the increased individual comfort, the diminution of individual suffering, and the banishment of all the most repulsive features of institutions set apart for the reception of human beings disqualified for ordinary life; but now placed amidst circumstances promotive in the utmost degree of their comfort, and in proportion to the possibilities, in each case, of mental amendment and recovery.

PART IV.

ABOLITION OF MECHANICAL RESTRAINTS AT HANWELL
IN 1839.

THESE pages are prepared for publication at a
time when no inducement exists, on my part, to
introduce matter of a merely personal nature, or
which does not appear to me likely to be of some
use to the reader. If, therefore, I now more
particularly allude to the subject of the Abolition
of Mechanical Restraints with reference to the
Hanwell Asylum, it is certainly with no design of
claiming for that institution, or for myself, more
than, or even so much as has been already accorded
by public opinion and the kindness of the medical
profession. But the change of treatment adopted
there seventeen years ago, and gradually effected,
including the entire disuse of restraints, having
been accomplished in the face of many difficulties,
all of which must be incidental to such an attempt,
wherever made, and the annual reports, in which

all the principles of the new system were successively laid down, and the progress of the experiment was carefully recorded, being now not to be procured, I think it most desirable to give some extracts from those made by me in the first seven years of that period, which may be regarded as having been peculiarly years of trial.

Although the phenomena of insanity and the character of asylums had occupied my mind for many years before I was appointed to the charge of the Middlesex asylum at Hanwell, in 1839, and the defective management of insane persons had been commented upon in a work published by me about ten years before assuming such duties, I was still deeply impressed with the responsibility of what I had undertaken, and my anxiety to avoid the abuses which I had freely condemned was largely mixed with solicitude as to the possible dangers to be incurred in the attempt in an asylum containing 800 patients. The perusal of Mr. Gardiner Hill's Lecture* had almost convinced me that what was reported as having been done at Lincoln might be accomplished in other and larger asylums. In the appendix to that lecture it appeared that Dr. Charlesworth, the physician

* A Lecture on the Management of Lunatic Asylums, &c. Delivered at the Mechanics' Institution, Lincoln, on the 21st of June, 1838, &c., &c. By Robert Gardiner Hill, M.R.C.S., and House Surgeon of the Lincoln Lunatic Asylum. Published April, 1839.

to the Lincoln asylum, had for sixteen or seventeen years been preparing the way for the non-restraint system by a vigilant attention to the effects of mechanical coercion, the instruments of which had been, by slow degrees, and in those long years, lessened in number at his representation, by the Lincoln Committee. A patient in that asylum had died in the year 1829, in consequence of being strapped to the bed in a strait-waistcoat during the night, and this accident had led to the establishment of an important rule, that whenever restraints were used in the night, an attendant should continue in the room; a rule which had also had the effect of much diminishing the supposed frequency of such restraint being necessary.

Various steps in the same direction had been recorded in the journals of the Lincoln asylum, and are especially alluded to in Mr. Hill's Appendix. Notice was required to be given of every instance of the application of restraints. Heavy iron hobbles and handcuffs were gathered together and destroyed. Strait-waistcoats were torn up. Dresses of a material not easily torn were provided for patients who generally destroyed their clothes. Bedding, in similar difficulties, was protected by strong coverings or cases. At length, in August, 1834, it was reported that for many successive days not one patient had been in mechanical restraint of any kind. At that time Mr. Hadwen

N

was the house-surgeon of the asylum. In 1835, Mr. Hadwen was succeeded by Mr. Gardiner Hill, who was soon able to say that not one patient had been in restraints, or confined to a room, in twenty-four days. In 1836, no instrument of restraint was used for three successive months; and at last, in 1837, Mr. Hill expressed his confident opinion that mechanical restraints might be altogether abolished. And thus the non-restraint system became established at Lincoln.

Much interested by these details, I devoted the few weeks intervening between my appointment to Hanwell and the commencement of my residence there in visiting several public asylums; in all of which, except in that of Lincoln, various modes of mechanical coercion continued to be employed. My visit to the Lincoln asylum (in May, 1839), and conversations and correspondence with Dr. Charlesworth and Mr. Gardiner Hill, as well as frequent communications with the late Mr. Serjeant Adams, at that time a member of the Hanwell Committee, and who had been much interested by the proceedings at Lincoln, more strongly inclined me to believe that mechanical restraints might be safely and advantageously abolished in an asylum of any size; and I commenced my duties as resident physician and superintendent of the Middlesex lunatic asylum at Hanwell, on the first day of June. In various asylums, some attention had been drawn to the subject of Mr. Hill's lecture; but I had observed that his views were received unfavourably, and sometimes in a spirit of hostility, or even of ridicule; and I found them by no means favourably regarded by the medical or other officers at Hanwell. The agitation, however, of so novel a question as that of abolishing instruments of restraint which, from time immemorial, had constituted a part of the daily treatment of numerous cases of insanity, had led, at Hanwell at least, to a somewhat less extravagant employment of coercive instruments than had before been common. After the first of July, when I required a daily return to be made to me of the number of patients restrained, there were never more than 18 so treated in one day—a number which would seem reasonably small, out of 800 patients, but for the facts that after the thirty-first of July the number so confined never exceeded eight; and after the twelfth of August never exceeded one; and that after the twentieth of September no restraints were employed at all.

The erection of the Hanwell asylum had, indeed, been a great step in the improvement of the condition of the pauper lunatics, not only of Middlesex, but of England; whose previous condition had been so wretched that the orderly arrangements of a large county asylum appeared to superficial observation matter not only of admiration, but of wonder. A commodious building, with extensive grounds about it, and gardens, and a farm in which several of the patients were employed, presented, indeed, a gratifying contrast to the dark and foul abodes in which the insane poor had so long languished, forgotten or unheeded.

When Colonel Clitherow and other benevolent persons in the Middlesex magistracy made preliminary inquiries into the actual condition of the pauper lunatics of the county, it was found that in the places in which they were kept, several were chained to the walls, in dirty and offensive rooms. Once a month a medical visit was accorded to them; and in the intervals they were left to the mercy of keepers. Before dusk, at the close of each dismal day, the patients were carefully chained in cribs; and on Sundays—a day of holiday to the keepers—the patients were not taken out of the cribs at all. Their Monday toilet, and probably that of every morning—except Sunday, when toilet there was none—was performed in a tub, in the yard, with the aid of a mop. The extravagance of soap was not permitted, and for 170 patients one towel was considered sufficient. The economy of this plan was evident, and the mortality attending it, although great, was not regarded. Horrible as these things were, they prevailed in some degree in every receptacle for pauper lunatics in England at that time. But all these old neglects were too easily forgotten; and it was therefore not a matter of surprise, or even of just condemnation, if a new county asylum, although in many respects faulty, was considered a model of perfection before unapproached. The building of such large structures at the expense of the county was so jealously watched, that its limited plan generally led to subsequent expenses of great amount, and when the asylum was opened a kind of necessity existed for concealing the real and unavoidable cost of maintenance. Thus a rigid economy, which had been the fatal vice of the older institutions and arrangements, and the fertile origin of much that was reprehensible, became an inherent part of the character of the new establishments.

The employment of the patients—now chiefly regarded as valuable in relation to its salutary influence on the patients themselves—was put too prominently forward as a source of pecuniary profit, whilst every item of expenditure was kept as low as practicable, to avoid the charge of unnecessary extravagance. This was the root of many evils, and several of these had naturally sprung from it, even at Hanwell. An inadequate number of attendants, engaged at low wages, and ill-qualified for their duties, became among the first consequences; and, as an inevitable result, the patients were neither properly superintended in the wards nor in the airing courts; at meals, nor during labour; nor at the hours of rising and going to bed. Disorders innumerable ensued; quarrels, and fightings, and injuries; and various accidents. Confusion often prevailed everywhere, and escapes were of frequent occurrence. The cleanliness of the patients could not receive proper attention; their clothing was defective, and even their diet was too scanty. Deficient ventilation, everywhere and always perceptible, and which rendered several portions of the building unpleasant by day, and most offensive by night, was a result of the same inattention which allowed almost countless panes of window-glass to be gradually replaced by squares of tin or of iron. Straw beds, with all their accompaniments of mice and vermin, were extensively used; and all the attentions required by patients unable to take care of themselves were lamentably wanting. And, what was especially objectionable to a medical observer, scarcely any proper arrangements existed for the sick. The infirmaries were ill placed, and wanting in every comfort.

Reviewing this state of things after so long an interval, I do not consider it as justifying any imputation of cruelty, or even of indifference, on the part of the management of the asylum. The small number of the attendants, their low wages, and consequent inefficiency, made a continual recourse to mechanical means of coercion and

security necessary; and over these means they had
unlicensed control. In some of the wards, especially
on the female side, the nurses were worse dressed
and wilder looking than the generality of the
patients; and the scenes daily witnessed were what
might be expected. Nor was it possible to effect
the diminution of restraints without attending, at
each step in the attempt, to some of the negligences
or deficiencies enumerated, and to which the easy
imposition of restraints had gradually led, and
which habit had confirmed. However humane the
officers, the amount of mechanical restraint could,
in such a general state of things, be reduced no
further. Its actual reduction had been less the
result of conviction than an effect of the pressure
of public opinion from without; and substitutes for
it had not been devised or adopted. The attempt,
therefore, to abolish restraints gradually and
entirely, made it imperative that all the evils for
the suppression of which restraints had been
habitually employed, must be met in some other
manner; and thus, in the minds of the officers
who resolved on this task, many resources originated,
and the ideas, one by one, of all those ameliorations
which, when put together, made the disuse of
mechanical coercion practicable, and constituted
the non-restraint system.

At the very commencement of these changes,
various circumstances, influential on the bodily

health of the patients, and secondarily on the
mind, received simultaneous and careful consideration from the committee of management. The
diet was made more liberal by an increase in the
proportion of solid food ; the ventilation of all
parts of the building was improved, and the number
of baths was increased. A considerable augmentation in the staff of attendants, their better
remuneration, and a more scrupulous selection of
them, created the required instruments in the hands
of the officers for carrying further improvements
into effect. Wards and airing-courts were no
longer permitted to be left without attendants ; and
order and regularity were everywhere enforced.
Quarrels were interrupted before words were
followed by blows ; and the mischievous habits of
patients rendered almost harmless by constant
superintendence, and prompt attention. Diligent
regard was paid to their clothing and bedding ; and
cleanliness was established and maintained to an
extent which at one time it seemed nearly hopeless
to expect. Those patients who were unable, or
even unwilling, to be employed, were regularly taken
out for daily exercise, and gloomy airing-courts
were converted into gardens. Recreations and
amusements were introduced for the benefit of the
listless and apathetic, as well as for those the
activity of whose minds required external means
of relief. Considerable alterations were made in

the religious services of the house; and it was required that the patients should attend the chapel neatly dressed. Prayer-books and hymn-books were furnished to them; psalmody was encouraged; and, by the appointment of a chaplain, two services were established on Sundays. Bibles, Testaments, and books of miscellaneous reading, were supplied to them under his direction and that of the physician, and the order of the chapel became much more rarely interrupted.

It was found very serviceable to institute various registers, which were required to be accurately kept; and also daily reports from each ward, by which means the state of each was made known at all times to the superintending physician, including the number of patients employed, or sick, or removed from ward to ward, or who had committed any injury or incurred any accident. No restraint and no seclusion of the patients was permitted without an immediate report being made of it. From that time the Hanwell asylum has every year furnished statistical information of great value, in tables first constructed with the kind assistance of Dr. Farr, of the Registrar-General's office, and also of the late Mr. Serjeant Adams.

These alterations could not have been carried into effect without the most zealous determination of the committee of management not only to improve the general treatment of the insane poor, but to carry the proposed system of non-restraint into full operation; supporting the physician, undismayed by misrepresentation and ill-grounded apprehensions of failure. Their task, as well as that of the physician, was for a time very difficult. The new system became, at one time, in consequence of circumstances which it would now be of no service to recall, the subject of great misapprehension and warm discussion among the magistrates at Clerkenwell, and even in the public papers. In the course of these events, the advocacy of the non-restraint system chiefly devolved on Mr. Tulk, on Mr. Serjeant Adams, and the late Dean of Carlisle (Dr. Hodgson), and was most ably maintained by them. Several notices of these proceedings are to be found in the *Lancet* during the year 1840. In the mean time, a reference to the records of events in the asylum in the years that had passed furnished irrefragable evidence that, when restraints were employed, outrages and accidents of every kind had been very frequent; and every month's experience confirmed the hope of those advantages arising from an altered system, which the experience of long years has now established beyond the possibility of contradiction.

It has recently been stated that Sir William Ellis, previous to his resignation of the office of physician in 1838, had effected much diminution in the frequency of resort to restraints. Of this neither the Reports nor the Case Books at Hanwell furnish, unfortunately, any particulars. Dr. Millingen succeeded Sir William Ellis; and, in the single year in which he held the office, the number of instruments of restraint in the asylum appeared to have been increased; and he subsequently professed his dislike of the non-restraint system very strongly,* The officers of the asylum who had been educated under Sir William Ellis were not among the supporters of the new system. They had not apparently partaken of his benevolent spirit; nor were they mindful of his precepts to be constantly and untiringly kind and watchful; and to persevere in affectionate attentions, day by day, and for weeks together, not discouraged by apparent failure, and confident of eventual reward.† His systematic employment of the patients, commenced at Wakefield, and more extensively carried out at Hanwell; his constant attempts to govern them by moral control; the pains taken, both by him and Lady Ellis, to diversify the life of the patients, and to procure them the solace of religious observances, should always be gratefully remembered. To do more than they effected, without the adoption of the non-restraint system, was, perhaps, impossible.

" It is due to the memory of the late Sir William

* Aphorisms on Insanity. By J. G. Millingen, M.D., 1840. P. 106.
† Treatise on Insanity. By Sir William Ellis. Introduction. 1838.

Ellis," says Samuel Tuke, in the introduction to the English translation of Jacobi's Work, " to bear in mind, that to him we are indebted for the first extensive and successful experiment to introduce labour systematically into our public asylums. He carried it out at Wakefield with a skill, vigour, and kindliness towards the patients, which were alike creditable to his understanding and his heart. He first proved that there was less danger of injury from putting the spade and the hoe into the hands of a large proportion of insane persons, than from shutting them up together in idleness, though under the guards of straps, strait-waistcoats, or chains. He subsequently introduced the system of labour at Hanwell; and now (1841) the same system has been carried out still more extensively in several of the asylums in Scotland." This change of treatment, therefore, constitutes a claim to the grateful remembrance of the name of Ellis; and although, in all cases of violent mania, he seems to have had recourse to restraints, he still wished and endeavoured to make the instruments of restraint as little painful as possible. For the old strait-waistcoat, which fastened the arms of the patient by long soft sleeves across the chest, or a-kimbo, he substituted wide canvas sleeves connected by a broad shoulder-strap, " so as to rest easily on the shoulders;" but by these sleeves the arms were fastened straight down on each side of the body, fastened with straps before and behind, whilst the hands were each placed in a tight bag of hard leather.* The sleeves were, in fact, as objectionable as any other mode of restraint, and equally productive of irritation, helplessness, dirtiness, and distress. The arm-chair recommended by Sir William Ellis, in which each arm of the patient was confined in " a padded box, which encloses the arm of the patient from a little below the elbow to the wrist," was not less objectionable ; and although he advised that such chairs should be provided with an apparatus for keeping the patients' feet warm in cold weather, it is scarcely necessary to say that this attention soon fell into desuetude. Attendants who fastened troublesome patients in chairs, cared nothing for such alleviations. In the part of Sir William Ellis's work devoted to the " Moral Treatment of Insanity," many passages occur which show his decided tendency to employ such treatment, to the exclusion of mere personal restraint ;† although he was still inclined to act on certain patients by exciting their fear, and by the infliction of electric shocks or the shower bath, or even the circular swing, as punishments.‡

When I began to reside in the asylum, a year after Sir William Ellis's residence there had ceased, the use of mechanical restraints was by no means limited to cases of violent mania. Instruments of

* Op. cit. p. 164. † Op. cit. 187, *et seq.* ‡ P. 227.

restraint, of one kind or other, were so abundant in the wards as to amount, when collected together, to about six hundred—half of these being leg-locks or handcuffs. The attendants had abused, as usual, the latitude of permission allowed them as to having recourse to such methods, and employed them for frivolous reasons, chiefly to save themselves trouble. On the female side of the asylum, alone, there were forty patients who were almost at all times in restraints; fourteen of these were generally in coercion chairs. All these patients were freed from restraints in September, 1839; and on a careful examination of thirty-seven of them, who remained in the asylum two years afterward, all were found improved in their conduct. Some, who had before been considered dangerous, were constantly employed ; and the rest were harmless and often cheerful.

The following extracts from my annual reports of the state of the asylum, made to the Committee, from 1839 to 1846, will show better, and more conveniently, and, perhaps, more instructively, the progress of the system of non-restraint at Hanwell in those seven successive years than any continued narrative. The Reports were drawn up from observation, in each year, of the facts related in them, until at length the experiment seemed complete, and the system established. I am enabled to refer to them with what I hope is a justifiable satisfaction, as I am not conscious of having, at any time, employed exaggerated expressions in them, or coloured any of the facts they contain too highly. In them, and in my " Clinical Lectures," published in the *Lancet* in 1846, and in my work on the " Construction and Government of Asylums," published in 1847, the inquirer into the subject of the general treatment of the insane will find the principal results of my experience. To these some future additions may possibly be added; but even as they at present appear, I trust there is nothing to lead the student into error, or to mislead the practitioner in this department of medicine.

FROM MY FIRST HANWELL REPORT (1839).

" The article of treatment in which the resident physician has thought it expedient to depart the most widely from the previous practice of the asylum has been that which relates to the personal *coercion* or forcible *restraint* of the refractory patients. Without any intention of derogating from the high character acquired by the asylum, it appeared to him that the advantage resulting from the degree of restraint permitted and customary in it, at the period of his appointment, was in no respect proportionable to the frequency of its application ; that the objections to the restraint actually employed were very serious ; and that it was in fact creative of many of the outrages and disorders, to repress which its application was commonly deemed indispensable ; and, consequently, directly opposed to the chief design of all treatment, the cure of the disease. The example of the Lincoln asylum, in which no patient has been put in restraint for nearly three years, came also powerfully in aid of an attempt to govern the asylum at Hanwell by mental restraint rather than by physical.

" Such an attempt could not be extended to all cases without some immediate inconveniences.

Attendants accustomed to rely on the easy help of close restraints, were reluctant to abandon them, and unexercised in the resources without which their abolition produced inconveniences, which they were not likely or able to compare with the remote evils produced by their continuance. Nor would the resident physician yet presume to say that strong restraint may never be required; but he begs to lay before the visiting magistrates a simple statement of the progress of an attempt to do without it. By a list of restraints appended to this report, it will be seen that the daily number in restraint was in July so reduced that there were sometimes only four, and never more than eighteen in restraint at one time; but that since the middle of August there has not been one patient in restraint on the female side of the house, and since the 21st of September not one on either side.

"There have, however, been occasional and brief instances of restraint, unsanctioned, in some cases, by the physician, and which do not appear in this table; but it correctly represents the total absence of continued restraint during the whole period since August 9th. For patients who take off or destroy their clothes, strong dresses are provided, secured round their waist by a leathern belt, fastened by a small lock. For some who destroy the collar and cuffs of their dresses with their teeth, a leathern binding to those parts of the

o

dress is found convenient. Varied contrivances are adopted, with variable results, for keeping clothing on those who would otherwise expose themselves to cold at night; and warm boots, fastened round the ankles by a small lock instead of a button or buckle, are sometimes a means of protecting the feet of those who will not lie down. As it is now and then necessary to confine the hands when a blister is applied, to prevent its removal; and as this, like all other temporary restraints applied with the justifiable plea of protection, is generally abused by being too much prolonged or unnecessarily severe, a kind of cape, as a covering for a blister, capable of being secured over it, has been thought of, and will no doubt be found practicable. Those who are in the habit of striking suddenly, tearing the bed-clothes, &c., sometimes wear a dress of which the sleeves terminate in a stuffed glove without divisions for the thumb and fingers. But no form of strait-waistcoat, no hand-straps, no leg-locks, nor any contrivance confining the trunk or limbs, or any of the muscles, is now in use. The coercion-chairs, about forty in number, have been altogether removed from the wards: no chair of this kind has been used for the purpose of restraint since the middle of August.

"It may be considered yet too early to pronounce a positive opinion on the general effects of these measures. In so large an asylum, filled with pauper lunatics, the means of mere mental control must always be limited, and the discontinuance of cruel restraints may only slowly be appreciated by the patients. But the resident physician is inclined to believe, after as careful observation at all hours as the space of a few months has permitted, and notwithstanding some peculiar difficulties, that the noise and disorder prevalent in some of the wards has already undergone diminution; that instances of frantic behaviour and ferocity are becoming less frequent; that the paroxysms of mania to which many of the patients are subject, are passed over with less outrage and difficulty; and that, if cases are yet seen which appear for a length of time to baffle all tranquillizing treatment, they chiefly, if not exclusively, occur in acute mania, the symptoms of which would be exasperated by severe coercion, or among those who, having been insane many years, have been repeatedly subjected to every variety of violent restraint.

" With respect to the discontinuance of the restraint-chairs, he may speak more confidently. Several patients formerly consigned to them, silent and stupid, and sinking into fatuity, may now be seen cheerfully moving about the wards or airing-courts; and there can be no question that they have been happily set free from a thraldom of which one constant and lamentable consequence was the acquisition of uncleanly habits.

" The substitution of mental control, implying constant superintendence, for physical coercion, has rendered it indispensable to increase the number of MALE AND FEMALE ATTENDANTS. Their former force was not only unequal to such an attempt being made with success, but quite inadequate to the preservation of that degree of order in the wards which the character of the asylum, the safety of its inmates, and even reasonable views of the advantage to be .derived from moral care, rendered essential. The wards were frequently left without keepers or nurses; the patients employed out-of-doors were in no responsible custody ; and accidents of various kinds were common.

" To maintain quiet and decent behaviour in the wards, airing-courts, grounds, and gardens at all hours ; to preserve the patients, many of whom are feeble and helpless, from various dangers, in all situations and seasons ; to prevent scenes of sudden violence, and put a stop to quarrels before abusive and irritating language leads to outrage ; to protect the weak, and exercise an habitual control over the powerful, the mischievous, and the destructive ; to guard the maniacal during the acute stages of their disorder, and to overpower the very violent without an unequal and dangerous struggle ; can only be effected when the attendants in an asylum are sufficiently numerous to ensure the extension of their superintendence to every part of the building or grounds in which the patients are employed, and the constant presence of at least one, but more generally of two, and sometimes of three attendants in each ward, according to its size and character. Without this provision, particularly in large wards, containing several patients who are occasionally violent, the most objectionable forms of restraint become necessary, and are yet insufficient to maintain peace or create security. Too severe an economy, perhaps more than any other cause, led to the prevalence of those extreme restraints in other establishments to which public attention has been at different periods so much directed. But physical restraint often fails to extend its effects beyond the body and the limbs; shouts and execrations attest its powerlessness over the excited brain; and the turbulence of the most refractory, thus uncontrolled or exaggerated, becomes a powerful obstacle to the well-doing of all the rest. No knowledge, no experience, no vigilance, no benevolence [in the heads of an establishment, can preserve the constant and perfect discipline required for the protection and cure of the insane, if their orders are not executed by an efficient body of intelligent, active, and watchful male and female attendants."

FROM MY SECOND REPORT (1840.)

" No event creates a more uncomfortable feeling
in the mind of the director of a lunatic asylum,
than the introduction of a patient apparently
determined on suicide.   In this large asylum,
several such cases are admitted in the course
of a year.   They generally come to us in merci-
less restraints, bound with cords, secured in any
manner within the reach of the terrified friends
and neighbours.   Nine suicidal cases are among
the admissions of the past year.   It affords gratification to the physician to be enabled to state, that
in all these cases means have been found to soothe
and comfort the minds of the patients, and,
apparently, to reconcile them to life.   Their
restraints have in all cases been immediately
removed, and in no case resorted to again.   They
have been watched, so long as it was deemed
necessary, during the day, placed in rooms with
other patients by night, and frequently visited.
Every instrument of danger, or obvious means
of self-destruction, has been kept out of their way;
and no measure likely to restore cheerfulness has
been omitted.   This is the general plan resorted
to.   But in almost every case of this kind the
bodily health is manifestly disordered; and when

proper remedial means are applied, the propensity to suicide is weakened, or disappears. Redness of the tongue; disinclination for food; irritable bowels; feebleness and emaciation; cold hands and feet; are not uncommon symptoms. In other cases a loaded tongue, obstinate constipation, and appearances of hepatic disorder, are observed. Both of these descriptions are chiefly applicable to patients between 40 and 50 years of age When submitted to proper remedial treatment, they commonly improve, although very slowly; the health being usually, or at least often, impaired beyond the hope of perfect restoration. It is impossible for attention to these patients to be too vigilant; but not at all impracticable to establish such systematic vigilance on the part of the officers and attendants as will afford security. To torment these unhappy patients with bodily restraints, would only fix the morbid determination more deeply in their minds.

" During the past year, not one instance has occurred, in which the resident physician has thought it advisable to resort to any of the forms of bodily coercion formerly employed. The use of the strait-waistcoat, the muff, the restraint-chair, and of every kind of strap and chain designed to restrain muscular motion, was discontinued on the 21st of September, 1839, and has never been resumed. The practice of fastening the epileptics, exceeding 100 in number, by one hand to their bedsteads at night, was gradually put an end to about the same period. After the liberation of some from this nightly restraint, the keepers and nurses, apparently satisfied with the results, discontinued the practice by degrees; and no inconveniences have followed, calculated to justify a return to it. In the intervals of their malady, some of the male epileptics are so reasonable as to be among the most industrious and best behaved patients in the asylum. This observation applies, although not to the same extent, to the female epileptics also; several of whom are young, and, except at the epileptic periods, mild and inoffensive in their manners. It was painful to behold sensible and well-behaved men, and harmless and delicate girls, not allowed to have the common privileges of rest at night, without one hand being strapped to the side of the bed, so as to prevent their lying with comfort either on the right side or on the left. The reasons assigned for this practice appeared to the resident physician to be perfectly unsatis- factory: and the practice itself rather dangerous than protective. Some epileptics spring out of bed during the fit; and for these very low beds are used; and sometimes a second mattress is placed by the side of the bed on the floor. During the day, notwithstanding the most watchful attendance, epileptics are liable to injury from falls, especially those who invariably fall on their face. But alert attendants very much limit these accidents.

" The management of the patients without bodily restraint has been applied to 1,008 lunatics, and has been acted upon for more than twelve months ; and it has thus far been found practicable to control every variety of case, without any fatal accident or serious outrage having occurred. For a time after perfect freedom of action was given to every patient in the asylum, some of those who were not accustomed to this indulgence abused it by breaking unprotected windows, and by tearing clothes and bedding ; but this destruction, which is known to be very great in asylums where restraint is much resorted to, has been much limited by contrivances which baffle the patient, without producing irritation. Even the stuffed gloves mentioned in the physician's last report as resorted to in some cases, in which the patients were accustomed to strike others, were found to possess so many of the disadvantages of restraint, that they were discontinued after a short trial. They were chiefly employed on the female side of the house ; and the report of the nurses concerning the patients to whom they were applied, as well as those who for the same reason perpetually wore leg-locks, is, that they are less combative and dangerous than they were before.

" Any contrivance which diminishes the necessity for vigilance, proves hurtful to the discipline of an asylum. Physical restraints, as they rendered all vigilance nearly superfluous, caused it to fall nearly into disuse; and, in proportion to the reliance placed upon them, innumerable evils of neglect crept in, which cannot exist where restraint is not permitted.

" Habitual intercourse with the insane cannot but impress those the most zealous for giving extended exercise for what is termed moral treatment, with the conviction, that the only prudent course with a lunatic during a state of violence, is to interfere as little as possible. Danger and mischief must, of course, be guarded against; but direct interruption is not always practicable; reasoning produces fresh irritation; contradiction commonly exasperates; and violence leads to injury, or leaves a lasting feeling of sullen resentment. Perfect calmness of demeanour and countenance, forbearance from sharp rebuke, the occasional inter-position of a soothing word, or of an idea that may divert the patient's thoughts, are not only the most useful measures at the time, but make some impression on the lunatic himself. A few broken expressions, in the midst of his violent talk, will sometimes indicate, to those accustomed to analyse such vehement language, that he knows what is said to him, and in what manner it is said. His

subsequent references to the interview often leave
no doubt of it.

"Sooner or later, calmer hours and days occur;
and it is in these intervals that all the resources of
moral management may be applied; and that the
practitioner must avail himself of the degree of
intelligence then manifested by the patient, and
of the remnant of the affections that survives.
Nothing must now be omitted that can have the
effect of gaining the patient's entire confidence.
On the accomplishment of this point everything,
in the future control of the case, turns.

"Among the obstacles to the acquisition of this
entire confidence, none is found practically to be
so great as any previous manifestation of anger,
or even of irritability. The imposition of severe
and immediate restraints, resorted to with such
feelings, and answering a mere temporary purpose
in a coarse mechanical manner, has a tendency to
render all the higher parts of treatment forgotten
in most cases, and in others difficult and impracticable. Lunatics, however audacious in aspect,
are generally the prey of fears and suspicions;
are prone to mistake the meaning of simple and
ordinary actions, and are easily agitated and
alarmed. They are only assured and rendered
attached by a continual course of kind and encouraging conduct, in which, even their keen and
distrustful observation can detect no real or

apparent unfriendliness, and no approach to deception. It can scarcely be necessary to remark, that any kind of cruelty is totally incompatible with such conduct on the part of those who undertake the treatment of lunatics; and even that severity, however occasional it may be, is fatal to its integrity. The reliance of the patient must be entire in order to be salutary. Whatever leads the patient to think himself deceived, encourages him to deceive, and there is no further dependence to be placed upon him.

" Misled by the lingering prejudices of great authorities, the resident physician for a time believed that cases in which it was judicious to assume a tone of severe displeasure and command, and to enforce obedience which persuasion had failed to effect, were of frequent occurrence. On reviewing instances of this kind calmly, he has always become convinced that patience, a little longer continued, would have been preferable. He has generally found the confidence of the patients for a time much shaken by violent attempts to control them; and it has sometimes only been regained after many weeks. Since the abandonment of the authoritative manner, except in very peculiar cases, (in which it requires to be employed with the utmost composure and appearance of solicitude), he has repeatedly found that violent patients may be persuaded to go into their rooms and be quiet, although half-a-dozen attendants would find it difficult to force them into such salutary seclusion. The success is greatest with those who have never been subjected to bodily restraints. In old mismanaged cases, the temper is rendered more irritable, and the mind more suspicious. Yet even in these inveterate examples, in which patients, long after coming to the asylum, have always appeared on the borders of frenzy, to which a word would drive them, the advantages of long continued gentle treatment have been at length plainly discernible. Each successive attendant upon such patients has assured the physician that no other kind of treatment has had any good effect upon them. The physician speaks from repeated observation, when he says, that no favourable impression could be made upon these patients, so long as restraints were either resorted to or threatened. Yet in these patients the mere mention of restraint was often observed to cause the patient's face to become deadly pale—an evidence of its efficacy as a punishment; standing quite apart from any proof of its efficacy as a means of moral control. The spectacle, in these cases, when the strait-waistcoat was determined upon, was most distressing. There was a violent struggle; the patient was overcome by main force; the limbs were secured by the attendants, with a tightness proportioned to the difficulty they had encountered ; and the patient was left, heated, irritated, mortified, and probably bruised and hurt, without one consoling word; left to scream, to shout, to execrate, and apparently to exhaust the whole soul in bitter and hateful expressions, and in curses too horrible for human ears.

" It was impossible to view these things, almost daily occurring, without resolving to endeavour to prevent them. Occasionally, peace was restored by the sudden and unexpected removal of the restraints; and at other times, restraints were allowed to remain on until the patient became quiet or sullen. In the first case, good was sometimes done ; in the second, none ever resulted. By degrees it was found that by refraining from restraint, although it was still alluded to, the patient felt that an obligation had been conferred ; and would promise good behaviour, and, for a short time, maintain it. But it was not until restraints had for many months ceased to be seen in the wards, that tranquil conduct of any duration was observed in these patients. Some of them have now proved capable of removal to the quieter parts of the Asylum ; after having been long considered the most hopeless patients in the house. Their malady is incurable; but it appears to have lost some aggravations resulting from years of mismanagement : for some of these patients are now middle-aged; became insane in the prime of life; and were sent here after being in many lunatic asylums.

" It seems desirable that the resident physician should take this opportunity of explaining the measures substituted for restraint at Hanwell; and the adoption of which, variously modified, is as important as the discontinuance of modes of treatment which had become perverted into means of habitual punishment. The physician is not anxious to dwell upon effects and general results which are open to the daily inspection of the visiting magistrates. To those who, more remote from the asylum, are liable to be influenced by vague reports of the manner in which it is conducted, the only answer to which none can take excception, must also be afforded by the general state of the asylum itself; always with this consideration, that a change of plan, involving the minutest as well as the most important parts of discipline, is only in progress, and not yet completed.

" SECLUSION.—All the substitutes for restraint are, like restraint itself, liable to be abused; but none can be made such instruments of cruelty by abuse. All are also liable to great misrepresentation: and none more so than that which is of all the most useful, the most simple, and the most approved of by the highest medical authorities— namely, seclusion. By seclusion is meant temporary protection of the maniac from the ordinary stimuli acting upon the senses in the refractory wards of a lunatic asylum. He is abstracted from noise, from the spectacle of a crowd of lunatics, from meeting those who are almost as violent as himself, and from every object likely to add to his irritation. But the mode in which seclusion is effected is also important to securing the benefits of it. If resorted to with violence, if accompanied with expressions of anger or contempt, if stigmatised as a punishment, and if followed by neglect, it may produce all the evil moral effects of restraint itself. If injudiciously persevered in in very recent cases, it exasperates instead of calming. The patient requires freedom of action; is relieved by strong muscular exercise; and this should be provided for by such a subdivision of airing courts as would leave one for the occasional use of a single patient, at least for a few hours in the day. After being indulged in active voluntary exercise for an hour, two hours, or such period as may seem desirable, the patient should be secluded. Calmness and sleep will sometimes follow, or sufficient tranquillity to enable the attendants and officers to talk to the patients with effect.

" Under the system of restraints, when a patient became noisy and violent, and particularly when some mischief had been committed by him, it was considered necessary, and it was the usual practice, to overpower him, and to put him in some kind of strait-waistcoat. This was done with great difficulty, and with much danger to the attendants. Observation has convinced the resident physician that this was a useless and even hurtful mode of management. It was like endeavouring to smother a fierce fire by heaping very combustible materials upon it. A maniac in the midst of his paroxysm, like a man in a violent fit of passion, should be interfered with as little as possible. The violence which, if met by violence, will become still more aggravated, will often, if left to itself, subside even in the course of five or ten minutes. Whatever the duration of the violent accession, its continuance is a bar to anything but such management as protects the patient and those about him. It is in intervals of calmness that the foundations of moral treatment must be laid, and the confidence of the patient gained. To acquire this confidence is the key-stone of all moral treatment; and nothing will so much oppose its acquisition as brutal or even impatient usage during the paroxysm.

" In the meantime, supposing the violent state to continue, the other patients should be removed from the neighbourhood of the one who is excited; all obvious means of mischief should be guarded against; and the attendants, although not directly interfering, should be watchful and ready. A soothing word now and then, or something new to

P

attract the attention, may be admissible ; but all with discretion. Supposing, as must often happen, that the violent fit does not immediately subside, and that the patient continues to vociferate, to swear, to abuse and threaten those about him, and to endeavour to strike them, something more must be done. But in this condition the worst thing that can be done is to struggle violently with him, to overpower him, and to mortify him by putting on bodily restraint. The only reasonable object of any treatment is to tranquillize the violent man ; and, of all modes of effecting this, surely violence is the most unreasonable. Seclusion effects the object more certainly than restraint, and without any violence at all. A lunatic is seldom, even in his most raving fits, insensible to what is said to him : he will often show, among his wildest and most extravagant expressions, that he is watchful of the conduct of those about him ; and when the ordinary observer would expect nothing from him but what indicated savage fury, those who are patient with him, and who, regardless of his wildness, continue to indicate their kind feelings towards him, will find that sometimes his voice falters, and his eyes fill with tears. These symptoms of emotion are very transient ; but they show that the sensibilities are not quite oppressed ; and they warn the practitioner, in language that ought not to be disregarded, to abstain from everything which can

further wound or oppress the feelings of an almost
ruined mind. These circumstances are now mentioned as bearing upon the manner in which the
seclusion of a violent patient should be effected.
Three or four attendants, possessed of courage and
good temper, should surround him; and telling him
that he would be much better if quiet, and in his
own room, should endeavour, by gentle occasional
efforts, to induce him to walk into it. It will
sometimes be found, that although he protests
loudly against the measure, his steps gradually
proceed in the direction required. At the same
time, steadiness and strength may be required
to prevent his retrograding; but well-qualified
attendants will not, on this account, resort to
violence. If he strikes or kicks them, they must,
of course, effect their purpose as speedily as possible, and with steadiness, and even with force;
but always without passion. As soon as the
patient is thus placed in his room, he is not
unfrequently found to become quiet, or if he
continues to talk loudly, it is not for a long period.
In all probability he will soon lie down on his bed,
and go to sleep. If he continues violent, he is at
all events out of harm's way. He will very seldom
attempt to hurt himself, and he can hurt no one
else. The window of his room should in all cases
be secured by an efficient shutter and lock. The
bedstead, which should be of wood, should be

fastened to the floor, and remote from the window. Sufficient light should be admitted through holes made in the window-shutter to enable the attendants, by looking through the inspection-plate in the door, frequently to ascertain the state of the patient.

" The abuse to which this seclusion is liable is that of being too prolonged. A troublesome patient being once locked up, it is natural that the attendants should have no very anxious desire to let him out: but if the superintendent is assisted by officers of proper activity, this abuse should be impossible. The seclusion should in all cases be immediately reported; and after two or three hours, some officer of the asylum should visit the patient, or at least look at him through the inspection-plate, so as to judge of the propriety of the seclusion being continued or put an end to. This should be done with great circumspection. If even the cover of the inspection-plate is moved roughly and noisily, the patient is roused and irritated. Still greater mischief may be done by prematurely going into his room. A daily report should be made to the Superintendent of the patients who have been in seclusion, and the number of hours they have been secluded. It is impossible to lay down rules for the general length of seclusion. Three hours, two hours, or one hour, in many cases answer every purpose. In other instances, after four or five hours, although the patient should be brought out, and a trial given of his capacity to behave well, it is not found practicable to have him at large among the other patients; and it is better to keep him in his room till the next day. Many patients liable to periodical excitement, and especially females, are far more comfortable if kept in seclusion during the whole period of their excitement.

" When the female patients are put in seclusion in consequence of any sudden outburst of passion, a very usual effect upon them is a vehement fit of crying and sobbing. In such cases, after a short interval, it is desirable that the patient should be talked to and soothed; and the seclusion should not be prolonged. If such a patient is neglected, seclusion will only produce sullenness. There are other cases in which a female patient, who would strike and kick those about her if at large, will become instantly quiet when put in seclusion; and, when seen through the inspection-plate, will seem so extremely tranquil, as to make it appear to those unacquainted with her, that she might be suffered to be at large without inconvenience : but if the door is incautiously opened, such a patient will be found to spring suddenly upon the intruder. The character of such patients becomes familiar to the attendants; but from perverseness, or obstinacy, they sometimes thwart the intention of the super-intendent by letting out the patient to astonish a visitor, or by prolonging the seclusion when they know it to be no longer necessary.

" In very young female patients, disposed to occasional violence, seclusion requires to be applied with peculiar precaution. The darkness appears to alarm them; and the solitude seems to aggravate the paroxysm. In all respects these patients require particular attention; the greater number of them being curable; yet so strongly affected, favourably or unfavourably, by all the circumstances around them, as easily to be rendered incurable by neglect or mismanagement.

" There are many patients subject to paroxysms of excitement of about a week's duration, who, of their own accord, will keep in their rooms at such a time; and who, although the door is not locked, will seldom offer to come out. There were no patients more injured by the imposition of restraint than these: the character of some of them, even during their most excited state, is improved since its discontinuance; and at other times, instead of being a terror to the attendants and the officers, they are among the most affectionate and grateful patients in the house.

" The resident physician dwells more minutely on seclusion, because he considers it as one of the most important of curative means, and as one of the least objectionable substitutes for every kind of restraint. It is open to no objection which is not doubly applicable to restraint. All the possible evils of seclusion were included among the innumerable evils of bodily coercion. Whilst the patients who were permitted to walk about in restraint were still capable of inflicting injury upon others, they were not protected from causes of irritation, or from the attacks of other patients. When put in seclusion, it was a seclusion which did not tranquillize. The arms or the hands were closely confined to the body ; or the arms, or the legs, were strapped or chained to the bedstead ; or the head was confined by a strap round the neck. In this state they were left for days or for weeks, in the most miserable condition in which a human being could be placed ; and often to the total ruin of all habits of cleanliness.

" It is of much consequence to observe that in whatever asylum it is determined to abolish physical restraints, several inconveniences must at first be experienced. There must be numerous adaptations to the new system. Under the restraint system, bad conduct is first permitted, and then punished: under the other, it is prevented. Under one system, coercion of the body is relied upon in every emergency : under the other, numerous resources must supply its place.

" The mere liberation from restraints, although it will prove a measure of extensive operation in a large asylum (concealed or slight habitual restraints

being generally numerous where severe restraints
are tolerated), is only a small part of the undertaking. The security and good behaviour of the
patients must then be placed in entire dependence
on the constant watchfulness and care of the
attendants; and a system of treatment be substituted for the restraint system, sustained by the
cheerful co-operation of every officer; so that the
whole government of the house may become kind,
protective, and, as it were, parental. For the
completion of such a plan, therefore, a united
household is indispensable. No one is qualified to
be an officer, a keeper, a nurse, or a servant in a
lunatic asylum in which such a plan is pursued,
who is not able and disposed to make every part of
personal conduct more or less conducive to one
great end—the comfort and cure of the lunatic
inmates. Their duties are peculiar, and require
peculiar dispositions, for the absence of which
nothing can compensate. No precepts or regulations can supply the want of those suggestions
which should spring from the heart.

" When restraints are to be discontinued, it may
be found, for the first time, that there is not a
room in the asylum properly adapted to the safe
keeping of a violent patient; not a window which
is not easily reached and opened; not a shutter
that can be properly secured; no ward door that
cannot be opened without a key, nor any clothes

or bedding that cannot easily be torn. The attendants may be too few in number; at once severe and slovenly; inefficient to the duties of guardianship devolving upon them, and unprepared either to prevent any accident, or to remedy any evil, when denied the support of restraint upon which they constantly leaned. The new system must also be much dependent for success, in a large institution, on the officers acting under the physician. Accustomed to witness all the abuses of restraint, and distrustful of other expedients, they may be prone to neglect other resources, and even the prompt application of remedial means, and their negligence will lessen the confidence and alacrity of the attendants. No superintendent, desirous to give the system an effectual trial, must be discouraged by these circumstances ; or even by finding that all his substitutes for restraint are, for a time, represented as more objectionable than restraint itself.

"One general error also seems to pervade the minds of those who most severely condemn the abolition of restraints: they always assume that if one kind of violence is discontinued, some other kind of violence must be substituted for it. It is scarcely possible to show by words the various means by which difficulties, the mere imagination of which alarms those not familiar with the insane, vanish before the patience, firmness, and ingenuity of officers who are determined that no difficulties shall be regarded as hopeless, until every effort has been tried. Those who are really interested in the subject and anxious to act upon the principle of non-restraint, should be witnesses of the instructive examples presented every day and night in institutions in which restraint is not resorted to.

"The resident physician cannot but repeat, as a circumstance requiring to be constantly guarded against, that officers and attendants who have been accustomed to rely upon restraints, are apt to exhibit an apathy and want of resources in difficulties ; and that their statements must be received with the utmost reserve. Patients who have sunk into a state of partial imbecility of mind, are well known to become utterly regardless of personal cleanliness ; and will sometimes swallow any kind of dirt and nastiness. Amidst the numerous and obvious means of preventing this, the attendants never think of any but one ; and that is restraint. Deny them the strait-waistcoat, and they let such cases take their chance. No decent precaution, no attempt to encourage cleanliness, no device for obviating what is disgusting, presents itself to their minds ; and a disposition may exist to represent such cases as illustrations of the wildness of the attempt to banish bodily coercion. In some very recent instances in this asylum, supplying these unhappy patients with a little bread

at bed-time, was resorted to by the resident
physician; and the patients have since been
reported as having relinquished the practice, previously represented in a manner calculated to give
him the greatest uneasiness."

FROM MY THIRD REPORT (1841).

" More than two years have now been completed
since the resident physician began to report to the
visiting justices the gradual disuse of mechanical
modes of restraint, and the substitution of a more
efficient superintendence by means of a greater
number of attendants of intelligence and respect-
ability; his motives, as then stated, were the
apparent inefficacy of mechanical restraint as a
means of preventing accidents and mischief; its
irritating effects on the violent; the alarm it
occasioned to the timid ; and its tendency to debase
those to whom it was applied, and to create
incurable habits of uncleanliness. The resident
physician gratefully remembers the consideration
these representations received from the visiting
justices in the autumn of 1839 ; and the kindness
and constancy with which his early efforts to abolish
a mode of treatment so objectionable were regarded
by them, in the midst of difficulties which he is
now happy to be able to refer to as entirely overcome.

" In October, 1840, after a year's experience,
made in circumstances some of which were
singularly unfavourable to the success of the

trial, he felt himself justified in announcing its probable success. Another year has now passed; and the experiment has for a part of the year been conducted by a united household. From the moment of this union of purpose among the officers and attendants, the obstacles besetting the experiment have diminished; accidents and assaults have become less frequent; and the general tranquillity and order of the asylum have increased. However unpleasant the recollection of the state of the asylum may be at the time of the commencement of the change of system, it affords the important knowledge that confusion among the patients is the concomitant of unfaithfulness in those on whose exertions the superintendent must depend, and the preservation of discipline easy when those whose office it is to preserve it are zealous and sincere.

" Every successive month appears to add to these encouraging effects; the attendants daily acquiring a clearer appreciation of a system from which violence of every kind is excluded. Its advantages are thus more effectually secured to patients newly admitted; and the general results strengthen the conviction that by abolishing restraints many other evils, considered inseparable from lunatic asylums, are at the same time swept away.

" In the course of the year, several patients have been admitted in restraints, and many more marked with restraints imposed before admission. The

management of all these cases has proved perfectly practicable without restraints.   In general,
the patients have seemed very sensible of the
benefits of their emancipation; and in some
instances in which patients so marked—marked,
indeed, for life—have recovered, they have delivered
a consistent and impressive relation of their former
treatment, and expressed their belief that it was
extremely injurious to them.   In one case, that of
a fine young man, of excellent temper (J. E.), both
ankles and both wrists were ulcerated, and he
informed us that this was done by handcuffs and
leg-locks, worn before admission ; and the whole
body so emaciated that he seemed to be sinking
fast into the grave.   For a short time this patient
was occasionally troublesome, and he was now and
then secluded : but he gradually became quiet in
his behaviour ; he grew stout, was employed in the
store-room ; and in four months went away, quite
well, and with the good wishes of all who knew
him.   This young man repeatedly said that he
owed his life to his removal to Hanwell.

" In another case (H. L.), a young man was
admitted whose back was covered with ulcers, and
he was apparently paralysed in his lower extremities.
He can now walk about ; and there is too much
reason to believe that the account given by his
relatives is correct, and that his ulcers, and the
temporary privation of the use of his lower limbs,

were occasioned by his having been long fastened down in bed, and consequently, as always happens when patients are so restrained, often lying on wet bedding.

" Very recently, a female patient (M. R.) was admitted, who was supposed to have lost the power of walking in consequence of paralysis : she is also gradually recovering, and walks about. Her friends report that she was always fastened down before she came to us. She proves to be perfectly harmless ; and, being an elderly woman, the use of her lower limbs would probably have soon been irrecoverably lost if she had not been removed.

" Great, and sometimes insuperable difficulty is experienced in attempting to gain the confidence of patients who have been treated with austerity, or subjected to restraints, before admission. They can scarcely be convinced that fair words conceal no guile, or that they will be allowed to sleep unbound. One patient (C. C.), a poor girl of 20, held out her hand a long time after going to bed for the first time at Hanwell, and could with difficulty be persuaded by the nurse that it would not be strapped to the side of the bed. She said she was accustomed to have one hand and both feet fastened at night. Her general demeanour proved to be remarkably quiet ; but now and then she was excited, and benefited by leeches, baths, and even by temporary seclusion. She now looks so stout and cheerful as scarcely to be recognised as the depressed creature who came to us in August; but she is still in a state requiring occasional medical treatment. On the same day, a stout, florid young Irish woman was admitted; very irascible; and loudly complaining of having been violently treated. There were marks of manacles on her wrists. In a few days her behaviour much improved. She soon became occupied in the laundry; and then a valuable helper in the kitchen of one of the officers; and in less than two months she left the asylum perfectly well.

" Cases of a somewhat similar description are too numerous for particular detail; and they are only alluded to as illustrating, by their subsequent course, the indiscriminate abuse of restraints of which the patients have been the unfortunate subjects. The importance of admitting patients of the poorer class as soon as possible into the asylum, when they become affected with insanity, cannot be overstated. Young persons are brought to us who have been a few weeks maniacal, and in consequence of the alarm or ignorance of those about them, have been locked up by the police, forcibly tied down in workhouses, exposed to severity and insult, and have had handcuffs put upon them, and been eventually sent to the asylum much exasperated by all that has passed. This was remarkably exemplified in a delicate young woman of 18, (M. S.), whose recovery commenced from the date of her admission, although she was both maniacal and disposed to suicide when she was first received; and who has left the asylum quite recovered. The wild gestures and frantic aspect of this young creature began to be lost when she had been two days in the wards. She became remarkable for mildness and amiability of conduct, but retained a strong recollection of the manner in which she had been treated before she was sent to us.

" To those who have opportunities of observing the extraordinary changes wrought in the most violent recent cases, by continual patience and kindness, it cannot but appear probable that some among the older patients, who remain immoveably sullen or morose, might have been benefited, at an earlier period, if they had not been treated roughly and without consideration.

" A prolonged maniacal attack is not unfrequently characterised by continual activity and a most ingenious disposition to mischief. When restraints were employed, these restless and troublesome patients were very frequent subjects of it. It prevented the necessity for the almost continual watching required, and which was too irksome to be borne by an attendant who could at once be relieved from his care by putting the patient's hands in a leather muff, or locking his ankles together, The inconveniences then created fell chiefly on the patient ; and many such patients were, by degrees, allowed to be either in constant or in very frequent restraint; always greatly to their detriment, and sometimes to their entire ruin. The patients now alluded to are seldom violent ; they are easily amused, and when amused are as playful as children : but they are irritable, and become uncertain in their temper under the annoyance of mechanical restraints. In the commencement of the attack, there is often evident bodily disorder, and it is one of the most serious of the evils attendant on bodily restraints that patients so treated do not receive that share of medical attention which they require. A strong illustration of this kind of case presented itself to the resident physician within the last three months.

" A male patient (R. E.) was admitted on the 23rd of June ; and reported to be ' dangerous to those about him.' It was avowed that in the asylum from whence he came he had been kept almost constantly in instrumental restraint for three months. He laboured under some religious and other delusions ; was almost always talking ; and somewhat restless in his habits ; so that although emaciated, and suffering from disorder of the stomach and bowels, it was not practicable to keep him among the quiet and feeble patients in the infirmary. He was placed, on that account, in a ward assigned to more troublesome patients, but he was of course never subjected to restraint; and, although fidgetty and always in action, he occasioned so little solicitude to attendants trained to habitual vigilance that he was never once even put in seclusion. A red and coated tongue, a voracious appetite, a disposition to swallow grass or gravel, frequent vomiting, irritable bowels, and a rapid pulse, afforded plainer indications for medical treatment than are usually met with in the insane; and clearly pointed out the case as one requiring remedial means rather than physical coercion. The state of the digestive organs became the subject of especial attention, and dictated a careful medicinal and dietetic treatment, under which this poor man has gradually recovered health and strength of body, and is fast advancing to the recovery of his mental faculties. In September he began to work in the garden. He is placed in one of the quietest wards; he writes affectionate and rational letters to his wife, and he lately partook of the sacrament in the chapel, at his own request.

"It is never possible for a physician to say of any case that it was treated on erroneous principles at a period anterior to that when his own observation of it commenced; but it is certainly difficult to conceive the necessity for mechanical restraints, and particularly for continual restraints, in a case of this description.

" T. F., a poor Irish labourer, was admitted in February last, looking wild and half starved. He had worn a strait-waistcoat, he said, in the workhouse from whence he came, and had been tied down in his bed. His mental disorder seemed the mere result of misery and starvation. The common comforts of the asylum composed him; he instantly began to recover, and is now perfectly well. He was placed in no kind of restraint or seclusion, but lodged in the infirmary and treated as a sick man. The excuse for dwelling on the value of attentions which every physician would consider both simple and obvious, is, that where restraints are at the constant command of the attendants, their ready imposition so entirely alters the aspect of the case that it scarcely gains the physician's attention at all.

" A female patient (S. P.) was admitted in January, labouring under complicated bodily disease, of which she died. The delirium which attended her malady had been thought indicative, before her admission, of the necessity of putting her into a strait-waistcoat. She had formerly been a nurse in this asylum, and told us that she helped those about her to put on the waistcoat, as they did not understand how to do it; a circumstance at least showing how little necessity there was for such an application. The frequent imposition of a strait-waistcoat on a submissive patient by a single attendant was one of the circumstances which originally awakened the attention of the resident physician to its habitual abuse.

" Incidents exemplifying the success attending the persevering application of diversified means to all kinds of cases, instead of restraint, are too frequent and too numerous to be reported. Thus (R. S. S.) labouring under acute mania, occasioned much trouble at night by his restlessness; various medicinal applications were tried without success, and his room and dress were so arranged, that his restless nights could be followed by no bad consequences on his health; but he was never fastened to his bed. At length it occurred to the house surgeon of the male side, that malt liquor sometimes proved an agreeable sedative. A bottle of Scotch ale was given to the patient at night, with the most satisfactory effects, and continued for some weeks; the quantity was then gradually reduced, but its omission for a single night was still followed by bad effects. During this time the patient, who had been reduced to the state of a skeleton, and was generally excessively noisy, has become fat, and in all respects greatly improved. He has been able to attend at chapel, and he sometimes plays the flute whilst other patients dance, and seems in good humour with everybody about him.

" Less striking cases were, however, among the more unhappy victims of restraints; restless, helpless creatures, seldom speaking, and seeming almost wholly stupid, and scarcely exciting attention. In a case of this kind (E. H.) a poor feeble man could not always be induced to lie down on his bed; he sometimes remained a great part of the night, or the whole of it, standing at the door as if ready to come out. He slept much by day, seemed well-nourished, seldom spoke, and never complained, but his ankles began to swell. Continued attention from the night-attendants and the keeper of the infirmary, together with a new kind of bed, in the course of adoption, instead of straw beds (and presently to be described), at length had the effect of habituating this patient to lie in his bed at night; and he may now often be seen by day, no longer sleeping, or stupid, or silent, but cleaning the knives and forks, polishing the fire-irons, and pointing to and telling of the result of his exertions, with much apparent satisfaction; and he appears in perfectly good health. It is unquestionable that if this poor man had been fastened in his bed by hand or foot, he would have become less and less capable of exertion, and that he would have soon entirely lost his health, and would also have remained in restraint every night until he died. The resident physician cannot forget having more than once discovered that dying patients were not released from restraints. Even in the restlessness of death, their feet were strapped or chained to the bedstead, and an order to liberate them seemed to occasion surprise.

" The resident physician feels himself called upon to speak of these subjects with less reserve than he has previously maintained, being assured that his efforts, and those of the visiting justices, to abolish useless coercion, would have met with no dissentient voice if the extent of its abuse had not been too considerately veiled. The certainty of abuse creeping on the use of coercion, whenever it is permitted, is an argument against it which nothing can overcome.

" The resident physician would earnestly impress upon all who may do him the honour to refer to his reports, with a desire either to form a judgment of the plan pursued at Hanwell, or an intention of adopting it, the necessity of considering *all its parts*, of which the discontinuance of mechanical restraints is only one. It is especially necessary to be guarded against the extravagant notions of *seclusion* set forth by the opponents of the non-restraint system. A reference to the report of last year, in which this very important particular of treatment was fully described, will show that, instead of being an imprisonment, productive of every moral and physical evil, it is a simple exclusion from the irritable brain of all external causes of additional irritation; that it places the patient in security, without fretting him by muscular bindings and impediment of limbs; that it secures other patients from danger, and the violent patient from injury when in restraint and defenceless, whilst it removes from his companions a spectacle always displeasing, and often alarming to them—that of a patient who, if at large, must be degraded by the muff or sleeves; that it very seldom fails to tranquillize the patient in a short time, and is even generally productive of immediate composure; that, with all this, it is easily effected, whereas the imposition of restraint was often only accomplished after a severe and irritating struggle, and was always most difficult when most required; and, lastly, that it has no general tendency to leave a revengeful feeling in the patient's mind.

" But to secure these advantages of seclusion, it must be remembered, that the term is applied to the temporary confinement of a lunatic in his own bed-room ; sometimes with the light partially excluded, sometimes almost entirely; that it must not be hastily resorted to; not carried into effect with anger, but steadily accomplished, when persuasion fails, by a sufficient number of attendants ; that it must not be accompanied with irritating expressions; nor applied as a punishment; nor unreasonably prolonged. All instances of seclusion should be promptly reported to the medical officer or matron ; the state of the patient in seclusion should be ascertained from time to time through the inspection-plate; and any appearance of contrition should be met with kindness. After half an hour, or one hour, or two hours, in different cases, the practicability of putting an end to the seclusion should be tried; except in instances where a longer repose of the brain is plainly required.

" This is the manner in which seclusion is directed to be practised at Hanwell; and although there are many days in the year in which there is not a single patient in seclusion during any part of the day, opportunities of witnessing its remarkable influence in inducing quietness are of course frequently afforded. In conducting visitors through the asylum, their attention is generally directed to the cases actually in seclusion, and whom they are commonly able to observe without occasioning them any disturbance.

" These advantages, there is every reason to think, were never derived from any form of mechanical restraint. The resident physician is aware that an opinion is entertained by a few respectable authorities that restraint exercises a salutary moral effect. He can recall no instance in which it seemed to him to do so. It has also been said that patients accustomed to violent attacks of mania, will beg to be put in restraints. He does not disbelieve this; but he has never met with an instance of it. He has occasionally known patients beg that restraints might be put on other patients:

he never knew them ask to have them put on themselves. He has met with one instance in which a patient, who recovered some years ago, states that when he was excited he always felt secure as soon as restraints were put on. The same individual, however, is now liable to attacks of excitement, but never solicits to be put in restraint of any kind. Patients liable to attacks of mania in a house where restraints are much employed, regard the accession of an attack with terror; but it is quite possible to screen them from every danger without restraint. The indignation of those on whom restraints were forcibly imposed; their eloquent exposition of its degrading and maddening effects; their fierceness when running about the wards in a strait-waistcoat; the alarm and discontent their presence occasioned to other patients; their speechless joy, their sobs and tears, when unexpectedly liberated, when both in seclusion and restraint, in the midst of a paroxysm of reproaches, prolonged until they were covered with perspiration and their lips were literally covered with foam,—are things of which the memory can never be effaced from the mind; and they make the ear deaf to specious representations of the comforts of straps and strait-waistcoats. When these results are contrasted with those of simple seclusion; when the anger, the ferocity, and sullenness, once characteristic of some of the wards in which restraints were habitually employed (as in the epileptic wards), are compared with the present indications of confidence and general good temper, the firm impression left is, that the general bad effects of restraint and its liability to abuse are immeasurably more pernicious than any thing that can be occasioned by its discontinuance.

"The quality of management which a careful superintendent will be continually learning in a lunatic asylum is *forbearance.* Scenes presenting at first sight an aspect of confusion and violence, are generally found to resolve themselves into simple elements if calmly surveyed for a few minutes. Furious gestures, threatening language, and abusive epithets, if not met by irritable and angry measures, commonly subside in a short time. Determinations of disobedience, apparently the most resolute, often yield to continued and calm persuasion. To all these events there are exceptions; but the exceptions will probably be always the least numerous with superintendents, officers, and attendants who preserve the most command over themselves. Firmness and determination may be even often required, but anger or passion always leave an uncomfortable impression that they have been at least superfluous. In these respects the resident physician has observed a considerable improvement in the ward-attendants since the disuse of restraints. The frequent imposition of hand-locks, or the muff, or the strait-waistcoat, or leg-locks—the difficulty with which they were put on a violent patient—the anger this imposition excited against the attendant, especially when put on, as was often the case, needlessly and unjustly, placed many of the patients and attendants in a state of continual hostility to one another. The attendant never spoke well of the patient, and the patient always complained of the attendant. At this time the patients in the refractory male wards are not unfrequently to be seen grouped round an attendant, who plays some instrument for their amusement; and patients, violent at other times, afford essential occasional protection to the attendant, when suddenly taken at disadvantage by some other violent patient. In the female refractory wards, the patients are usually found either assembled round a work-table with the nurses, or sitting by them on benches in the airing court, or riding with them on the rocking-horses. In both the male and female wards there is an appearance of a good feeling between the patients and attendants; and when it is necessary to use some force, either to insure seclusion or to administer a bath, it is done after long attempts at persuasion, with a quietness, promptness, and efficacy, by which the patient is taken by surprise, and obedience ensured without anything being done which gives the patient much offence.

" RELIGIOUS SERVICES.—It affords the resident physician much satisfaction to be able to say that the kind and judicious co-operation of the Chaplain, and his frequent and unreserved communications, are such as to inspire him with the fullest confidence that the ministerial offices performed in the asylum are carefully adapted to patients so peculiarly afflicted ; and administered in a spirit so temperate, earnest, and sincere, as to extend their benefits to every case in which prudence can permit a trial. Long experience can alone determine the cases to which religious attentions are applicable : they are sometimes beneficial where advantage was scarcely hoped for, and sometimes excite when no excitement was expected. They are also not equally applicable to the same patient at all times. Nothing can meet the various difficulties incidental to such delicate trials, except the constant and confidential communications of the physician and chaplain to each other. If the physician may sometimes prevent mischief that might arise from an ill-timed religious appeal, the chaplain is sometimes enabled by his intercourse with the patients to demonstrate that the influence of his spiritual conversation is deeper and more permanent than the physician might expect. By their continual co-operation alone can the zeal, judgment, and experience of both be so combined and directed as to throw light on a subject which, independently of its serious importance in a religious point of view, is connected with the interesting psychological question of how far the feelings and understanding may act and be acted upon in the various shades of mental disorder ;—how far, when the mental state disqualifies for worldly duties and pursuits, the affections and the vestiges of reason enable the afflicted lunatic to look up to his Creator. Experiments in relation to this important subject do not yet appear to have been made on a sufficiently extensive scale either to justify enthusiasm or despondency. It is not improbable that future reports may contain some interesting particulars relative to a subject on which at present very little seems to be known.

" Like every other part of a system that appeals to what remains of the reason and the feelings, a perfect trial of what could be effected by spiritual means was incompatible with modes of treatment which produced gloom, discontent, or ferocity. The ordinary public services at Hanwell were much more liable to interruption before the disuse of mechanical restraints ; and on looking back to the instances of disturbance which then occurred, it is curious as well as instructive to remember, that the patients who interrupted the services by noise or violence were almost always such as had been the especial subjects of mechanical restraint. At that time Sunday was a day of more than usual anxiety ; whereas there is now no day in which the aspect of the whole asylum is more tranquil and comfortable. The attendants and the patients assemble for chapel neatly dressed ; the congregation is usually about 300 ; and when the services are concluded, the patients may be seen walking down the galleries which lead from the chapel, as orderly as any crowd in a churchway path. Although they have no work to occupy them on Sundays, they may be seen sitting composedly in their wards after the service, or taking their dinners with every appearance of order and comfort. All such general descriptions are liable to occasional exceptions. One noisy patient may disturb fifty patients ; and the paroxysms of mania may occur on Sunday as on any other day ; but the general character of the house on Sundays is certainly such as is above described."

FROM MY FOURTH REPORT (1842).

" The annual reports presented by the resident
physician in 1839, 1840, and 1841, contain the
details of a plan adopted by him from the Lincoln
asylum, and persevered in, with such modifications
as experience suggested, with the sanction of the
visiting justices, to dispense, in the treatment of
the insane, with all the ancient bodily restraints.
The difficulties attending the commencement of the
undertaking, its progress, and its eventual success,
have been already related in those reports without
disguise, and, it is believed, without exaggeration.
The resident physician has now but the agreeable
task of recording, that time, and patience, and the
zealous co-operation of all the officers of the
asylum, have enabled him to overcome many
obstacles, and have confirmed him in a belief, at
first encouraged with much diffidence, but now
established beyond the likelihood of ever being
overthrown, that the management of a large asylum
is not only practicable without the application of
bodily coercion to the patients, but that, after the
total disuse of such a method of control, the whole
character of an asylum undergoes a gradual and
beneficial change.

" A long indisposition, attended with a mor-

tifying interruption of your physician's active
duties, has, by converting him into little more than
a spectator of what was taking place, at least
enabled him to exercise the calmer observation of a
bystander ; and his return to the asylum, after the
absence accorded to him by the kindness of the
visiting justices for the recovery of his health, gave
him an opportunity, by the strong impressions
incidental to a return to so extraordinary a scene,
to appreciate, perhaps more justly than he could
otherwise have done, the general results of a system
now three years in undisturbed operation, excluding,
as much as possible, every cause of physical and
mental uneasiness.   The appearance and general
state of the patients in the wards, or when taking
exercise ; when engaged with in-door amusements,
or when assembled at dinner or supper ; when at
work in the various departments of industry
connected with the institution, or when attending
divine service ; the order, activity, and cheerfulness,
pervading the asylum by day, and the tranquillity of
the whole house by night, are all indications that
the general management of so many disordered
minds is productive of those salutary effects which
are the object of all management.

"The impression produced on patients newly
admitted to the asylum is also strongly indicative
of the general character of the place being favourable to curative endeavours.   Their wildness and

irregularities often rapidly subside, and their habits conform to the general order and the decorous routine so remarkable in the majority of their fellow-patients. The continued operation of a tranquillizing system has produced effects even on the character and manners, and, as it would seem, on the disposition of not a few of the old and incurable patients; several of whom, formerly accustomed to meet the officers with endless complaints, seem now to have lost their fretfulness, and to be satisfied and content. Accidents, anxieties, and agitations must always be incidental to any house in which all forms and varieties of mental disturbance and disease are accumulated; but the resident physician believes that all the officers of asylums who are experienced in both methods of treatment, have found, or will find, that the liberation of their patients from restraints has lessened the frequency of accidents, and diminished the anxieties and agitations of those having the charge of them; so that even the various contrivances at first required for the prevention of evils and inconveniences formerly opposed by restraints, as strong dresses, seclusions, and window-guards, become less required.

" It continues occasionally to happen that patients are brought to the asylum in severe restraints. These are invariably removed at once, and they are never put on again; yet, from this immediate and systematic liberation, not one important accident, scarcely any inconvenience, has arisen. Every admission more strongly manifests the importance of regulating all the circumstances connected with the arrival and reception of a patient, with a strict regard to reconciling the new comer to the asylum. The only instance during the last year in which the attendants were set at open defiance, and one of them was severely hurt by a patient just received, occurred in the instance of a male patient, who was so quiet before his arrival that he had been entrusted to drive the carriage which conveyed him and others during a part of the journey; but he had been told that the other patients only were to remain, and on discovering this foolish deception, he became for a day or two unruly. He afterward behaved extremely well.

" The state of mind of a patient of ordinary sensibility, on arriving at the gates of a lunatic asylum, is usually somewhat agitated. It is then, amidst the fears and distress of the sufferer, to whom all is new and strange, that confidence is to be gained, and the first steps of successful moral treatment are to be taken. The manner in which new patients are addressed, the attendants to whom they are confided, the personal interest taken in them by the officers, the wards in which they are placed, the employment assigned to them, are all matters of great consequence; not only as allaying immediate anguish in many cases, but as exercising an influence over every curable patient from the hour of reception to the hour in which they leave the asylum.

"There are yet too many cases in which this kind and rational plan derives advantage from the injudicious severities to which the patients have been subjected before their removal. Cases illustrative of this have been spoken of in former reports. Among the patients discharged during the present year, H. B., a man who had been a respectable innkeeper, alluded, on quitting the asylum after his recovery, to the manner in which he had been received when he came to it; and he declared that, for nearly three previous years, he had never had a kind word addressed to him, until, on the day of his arrival at Hanwell, he had a conversation with one of the officers. He had remained eleven months in the asylum, and had passed through several attacks of recurring maniacal excitement, but the impression of that first conversation had never been forgotten.

"J. J., a middle-aged woman, was brought to the asylum in a strait-waistcoat in May last. Her spirits were greatly depressed; she had attempted to destroy herself; but she was perfectly tranquil, and spoke rationally. When the strait-waistcoat was removed, and she was talked to in a cheerful and encouraging manner, her countenance completely changed, and hope was evidently revived. In a few days she was busily employed and content, and she gradually got quite well.

" Another female patient (M. B.) evinced the liveliest surprise on being conducted with common civility to a decent bed-room, declaring that in an asylum from which she had been brought, the nurses treated her without any respect, dragged her day clothes rudely off, and left her to lie on straw, scantily covered with a rug. Although a woman of the poorest class, she keenly estimated the difference in her treatment, and often spoke of it. In a few months she left the asylum, perfectly recovered.

" There is, however, great reason to hope that the injudicious practices above alluded to, by which the early and most important period of the malady is too often wasted, will soon be entirely unknown in all asylums, public and private. The reports of many public asylums contain statements and observations strongly indicative of a general and progressive improvement, directed by an increasing conviction, confirmed by all intimate experience with insane persons, that in a large majority of cases of insanity the powers of observation are active, and the understanding has a considerable range of exercise; whilst the affections exist as warmly, and the sensibility is as acute as in a state of perfect mental health. Instead, therefore, of the majority of insane persons being now consigned to the chances of cruelty or oblivion, the utmost care is taken to act on what remains of intellect and feeling in each case; so as to direct the impaired faculties of the understanding, if not always usefully, at least safely, and at the same time to cherish and govern the affections by all the resources of compassionate protection. Such, unquestionably, are the general principles by which the treatment of the insane is regulated at the present period, variously carried into effect in various asylums. The results are daily developing themselves to all daily observers, and can scarcely yet be fully known and appreciated; but every year is affording new and satisfactory proofs that the principles are not dangerous or delusive, but founded in reason and fertile in advantages. Neglect and disregard, violence and intimidation, aided by all the devices of mechanical restraints, are everywhere disappearing; and everywhere, as they disappear, the application of all the powers and influences of sound mind to the recovery of mind impaired takes the place of them. The consequences may not be that a much greater number of perfect recoveries are effected—for recovery is impossible in a majority of cases of insanity—but the actual number of the insane thus kept in the living and intellectual world, and enjoying a great share of happiness, is immensely increased.

"Insanity, thus treated, undergoes great if not unexpected modifications; and the wards of lunatic asylums no longer illustrate the harrowing description of their former state. Mania, not exasperated by severity, and melancholia, not deepened by the want of all ordinary consolations, lose the exaggerated character in which they were formerly beheld. Hope takes the place of fear, serenity is substituted for discontent, and the mind is left in a condition favourable to every impression likely to call forth salutary efforts. A chance is thus afforded, to every impaired mind, of recovery to an extent only limited by causes which no human art can remove."

FROM MY FIFTH REPORT (1843).

" The whole experience of the last twelve months has fully confirmed the impression, made in the years preceding, that by the abolition of physical restraints, the general management of the insane has been freed from many difficulties, and their recovery in various degrees greatly promoted. Fresh illustrations have been daily afforded of the advantage of those general principles of treatment which have been expressed in former reports ; and of which the effects are to remove, as far as possible, all causes of irritation and excitement from the irritable ; to soothe, encourage, and comfort the depressed ; to repress the violent by methods which leave no ill effect on the temper, and leave no painful recollections in the memory ; and, in all cases, to seize all opportunities of promoting a restoration of the healthy exercise of the understanding and of the affections.

" Every separate article of treatment, every prescription, every direction, has these objects more or less immediately in view ; and the full results of this general system, wherever it is allowed to be consistently followed, and, as a consequence, to be at once, and from the beginning, applied to all

new cases, and perseveringly and uniformly adapted
to the older and more confirmed, will be more
perceptible every year; chiefly, and at first, in
large asylums, containing numerous patients long
affected with mental disorder, but eventually in
every house in which even a single insane patient
is the object of particular care.

" INSTRUCTION OF THE PATIENTS.—The classes
for the patients have been in operation only
a few months.   Each class consists of ten or
fifteen patients, and no class is occupied for
more than one hour at a time.   Among the readers
may be seen some who were formerly looked upon
as among the most troublesome patients in the
asylum, and several who are liable to occasional
attacks of maniacal excitement; but they attend
the classes with gratification, and observe a remarkable order and decorum; reading each a verse or
portion of a page in turn, with attention and
correctness.   The articulation of some of these
readers is impaired by their malady, but several
read with an earnest expression which is peculiarly
impressive, but difficult to describe.   The greater
number of the readers hitherto assembled have
been those who had learned to read in former years;
but of these several had lost the habit of reading,
and have much improved by practice.   Their
power of application, and their memory of the
previous day's lesson, have been observed to become

strengthened by these daily but not long-continued habits of attention. The teachers, and particularly the schoolmaster, have had the disadvantage of endeavouring to teach those who are for the most part incapable of employment, and, as may be inferred from that circumstance, the least capable of profiting by their instructions.

" Writing has been taught to some who were previously unable to hold a pen. Others who had formerly learned to write, were found to have forgotten the art, and required to begin again. It has often been observed that on the first day of going to the writing-class, the patients would scrawl over the page quite irregularly ; on the second day they would try to imitate the copy ; and in a few days write with care. They take particular pleasure in this acquirement, and exhibit their copy-books with much satisfaction. One female patient, who was thought to be too excited for the class-room, almost forced her way into it on one occasion, and when there wrote a copy with more than usual carefulness ; this patient, a married woman of forty, had not learned to write before she came to the asylum. Her application is often interrupted by grievous attacks of illness ; but in her happier intervals writing is her solace, and she has of her own accord written hymns from memory. Another female patient, who had never been taught to write before, and now writes very carefully, was formerly almost always in restraint. Singular difficulty is found in teaching these scholars to form each separate letter in cases in which there has never been any previous instruction; but the difficulty is surmounted by patience in the teacher, and anxious care in the learners. Some variety has been imparted to the occupations of the class-rooms by occasional descriptions of different parts of the earth, aided by reference to maps and to a globe; and in the classes for the male patients simple descriptions of various animals with pictorial illustrations have been found to excite a lively interest. Drawing and singing have agreeably occupied a few of them ; and a class of arithmetic has been formed on the male side.

" The patients assemble cheerfully, go through the little that is required of them without impatience, and seem to be very sensible of the comfort of the quiet occupations of the schoolroom, and to derive much pleasure and some advantage from efforts revived, in some instances, after long disuse, and awakened in others for the first time.

The resident physician is desirous not to exaggerate the immediate or the prospective advantages of this attempt to educate the insane poor. If the occupations associated with it are considered as little more serviceable than amusements, they may be still deserving of attention. If their results among the poor and uninformed should never be great, greater consequences may follow among patients of a different class; and in this instance, as in others, the example of so large an institution as Hanwell may be deeply felt, far beyond the limits of the immediate regulations of the Middlesex Asylum. The short trial already made has at least been attended with no obvious inconvenience; and it has not been permitted to interfere with the ordinary occupations of the asylum. The plan has been applied to about 80 of the female and to more than 120 of the male patients, and in no instance has attendance at the classes been compulsory.

" Among the inducements to persevere in this attempt, may be mentioned the more advantageous state in which the chaplain is disposed to think it may place the patients as respects the capability of receiving and profiting by religious instruction; which is found, as may readily be supposed, to be much impaired by the torpor and inactivity of mind so generally incidental to their disease."

FROM MY SIXTH REPORT (1844).

" Five years having now been completed since the abolition of the use of the strait-waistcoat, the muff, the leg-locks and handcuffs, the restraint chair, and every other form of mechanical restraint in the asylum, without the occurrence of any accident which the ordinary application of such modes of restraint could have prevented, and with a marked improvement in the character of those parts of the asylum in which they were in continual use, I should not think it necessary to say more on this subject than that my confidence in the practicability, safety, and advantages of the non-restraint system has gained strength by every year's experience since September, 1839, if I did not observe that much misconception still exists concerning the substitutes for restraints, in consequence of which doubts continue to be entertained, by many whose opinions must always have considerable weight, respecting the real advantage of this mode of treatment.

" The principal error is that of confounding the idea of temporary seclusion in ordinary sleeping rooms with solitary confinement.

" Seclusion, as directed to be practised at Hanwell, is but the removal of a patient from a gallery to a quiet bed-room opening directly out of the gallery; from noise and excitement to tranquillity. It is only resorted to when the patient cannot be at large with safety to himself or to others, and when he is not in a state to be influenced by persuasion or conciliated by kindness; and it is only continued until the temporary passion has subsided and the danger is past. In extreme cases, the protection of the patient is further secured by his being placed in a room of which the floor is a bed, and the four walls are padded. The room is not always darkened even by the closure of the shutter, and it is never completely dark. The seclusion is immediately reported to the medical officers, and a daily record of every seclusion is kept, even in cases in which it is only continued for half an hour, or for a shorter period.

" There is no single point in the management of the patients at Hanwell to which I have paid such frequent and anxious attention as to seclusion and its effects, immediate and remote. Its immediate effect is, of course, to protect the other patients, or the patient himself, from every danger: but it also scarcely ever fails to calm the patient's feelings, and to put a stop to his vociferations almost as soon as it is carried into effect. The patient who was five minutes before filling the gallery or the air with shouts, and exhausting himself in vehement and menacing actions, is found at once to cease to shout and threaten; to walk up and down his room, quickly at first, but soon more quietly; then to sit down and read, or to lie down and sleep. Women so secluded will walk about for a short time, and then take up a needle and thread and begin to sew. These effects of seclusion I continually observe; and the exceptions to them are most rare.

" The subsequent effects of seclusion are not less valuable or important. On being liberated from seclusion the patient's temper is not impaired. The seclusion and its consequences produce no bad effects on the other patients. It has neither alarmed nor offended them: they even appreciate its necessity, and it may almost be said its comfort to all parties.

" It is to be ascribed to want of opportunities of observation that such a simple exclusion of irritations from an irritable mind, an exclusion not found to be necessary in more than four or five instances in any one day in the year among a thousand patients, and seldom prolonged beyond four or five hours in any of those instances, during which time the patient's state is frequently ascertained by means of the inspection-plate in the door of his room, and all his reasonable wants and wishes are attended to, should ever have been confounded with the idea of solitary confinement—the latter in reality comprehending a privation of almost all the stimuli upon which the integrity of intellectual and physical life depends.

" Not one of the advantages derived from seclusion is compatible with the use of mechanical restraints. When *combined* with seclusion, which they frequently were under the restraint system, they even appeared to neutralize all its good effects. They are either imposed easily, and then without any necessity, or to repress extreme violence, and then with violent resistance and a struggle in which injuries are exchanged. They irritate, and heat, and disorder the body, and degrade and exasperate or subdue the mind. They induce an entire contempt for or neglect of all remedial means. They lead of necessity to dirty habits, and withal fail in a general way to produce tranquillity: the tongue remaining free to express the bitterest feelings and curses of an outraged maniac. Against sudden outbreaks of violence they constitute no protection, unless perpetually imposed, which none of the advocates of restraint would wish them to be. When once imposed, their use is almost always prolonged beyond necessity, and becomes repeatedly and wantonly resorted to. The officers and attendants who act with such aid become habitually cruel; they think of punishing the patients, not of curing them; and the patients, frequently and often unjustly put into restraint, become morose and revengeful. Many of their companions become distressed and irritated by beholding frequent scenes of violence, and the character of the asylum becomes changed and dangerous.*

" It is to be remembered, too, that nearly all the terrible accidents for the preservation from which mechanical restraints are held up as essential, have taken place in asylums in which they have been and continue to be used and abused. Even the accounts given of such accidents by those who adduce them as arguments for restraint prove that the accidents arose from negligence, or the want of that superintendence without which restraint is unquestionably necessary. From a sudden and fatal blow no possible extent of restraint can afford continual protection. There is great reason for believing that a disposition to commit suicide prevails most, and becomes most inveterate where restraints are most employed ; and is even created in many cases by their use. That when habitually or frequently endured they lower the whole character is proved by all experience ; and I believe that in asylums in which they are never resorted to, the patients are rarely if ever found to inflict injuries on themselves ;

* In support of these observations I need only refer to the account of restraints as now practised in some parts of England, contained in the late " Report of the Commissioners in Lunacy" to the Lord Chancellor. Pages 43, 48, 53, 54, 55, 58, 59, 60–63, 73. It is scarcely possible to conceive more forcible illustrations of all the immediate evils that arise from them. But the remote consequences are also numerous, and scarcely less dreadful.

whilst the impressive testimony of some of the sufferers is not wanting to show that their coercion cherished every wild and dreadful fancy, and every inordinate and depraved propensity. It seems, indeed, impossible to devise anything which so effectually excludes its victims from all moral or religious influences.

"I entertain no doubt that if those who yet question the propriety or safety of entirely disusing mechanical restraint were constantly living in asylums, and enabled to watch the effects of the two modes of treatment from hour to hour and from day to day, their doubts of the expediency of the non-restraint system would soon be entirely removed. It is at least worthy of especial observation that nearly all the strongest supporters of the non-restraint system reside in asylums, in the midst of lunatics ; and that very few of its opponents do so ; and that no attempt to dispense with the use of restraints in any asylum has been finally abandoned as unsuccessful.

"An intimate acquaintance with the patients at Hanwell enables me to bear testimony to the improvement observable in the character of many of the older patients since all the instruments of coercion have disappeared, and all the violence that belonged to the coercive system. There are yet patients in the asylum who bear on their arms and legs the ineffaceable marks of bonds of iron and cord, and whose narratives, from their own lips, show too plainly how far every feeling of humanity was forgotten when restraints were a part of the regular treatment of the insane.   The general state of the asylum, and the infrequency of seclusion, strengthen the conviction that the old restraints were superfluous; and patients are to be seen in it in the recent stage of mania, in its most lively and acute form, and for a considerable period, yet preserving a character of good humour, and of trust and confidence in those about them, which are highly favourable to their progress and recovery.

" In former reports I have described some of the substitutes for restraints successfully employed in the Hanwell asylum; as various dresses of strong materials, blankets protected by a strong covering, and padded rooms.   Continued experience has proved that these means, and a watchful and kind superintendence, amply suffice to meet all the ordinary and extraordinary inconveniences and difficulties of cases of insanity; to check destructive and uncleanly habits, and to protect patients from injury.   Even the strong dresses, blanket cases, and padded rooms become less frequently in requisition in proportion to the continued influence of another substitute for restraint, and one the chief of all, although not enumerated by the best writers who have lately endeavoured to weigh and compare the merits of the new and old systems of treatment. A knowledge of the prejudices in favour of any restraint that ensures secresy in cases of insanity occurring in private families; of the universal leaning to it in private asylums;* and of the obstacles yet existing in the way of its entire abolition in some public institutions makes me anxious to take this opportunity of expressing myself distinctly and publicly on this very important practical point.

"I have always endeavoured to enforce as a principle essential to the success, or even to the existence of the non-restraint system, properly so called, a constant and uniform application of all the resources of kindness and humanity, and a constant regard to the recovery attainable in each case. This can only be effected by means of well chosen, well-trained, and well governed attendants, under the direction of medical officers qualified by their education and enabled by their position in the asylum to devote their minds calmly and usefully to the protection of the insane, and to ensuring their general comfort, even where a cure is hopeless. By the services of such attendants and officers the patients may be won to salutary occupations, supplied with well devised amusements, and fur-

---

* "In all the houses receiving private patients, restraint is considered to be occasionally necessary."—*Report of the Commissioners of Lunacy*, 1844, p. 154.

nished with instruction suited to their impaired faculties.

" Where these conditions do not exist, or are not complete; where the attendants are inefficient or ill-taught, or the medical officers without proper authority, the system of non-restraint must be imperfect, and rest on an insecure foundation. The strait-waistcoat may not at once re-appear; but severity will only have quitted one shape to put on another : no uniformity of system will prevail; the patients will be exposed to regulations resulting from caprice or suggested by opposition; remissness will ensue ; accidents will occur and be ascribed to the system which really arise from its neglect; severity will follow, and the retaliations which follow severity ; and every thing will tend to the restoration of mechanical restraint.

" But, after five years' experience, I have no hesitation in recording my opinion, that with a well constituted governing body, animated by philanthropy, directed by intelligence, and acting by means of proper officers, entrusted with a due degree of authority over attendants properly selected and capable of exercising an efficient superintendence over the patients, there is no asylum in the world in which all mechanical restraints may not be abolished, not only with perfect safety, but with incalculable advantage."

FROM MY SEVENTH REPORT (1845).

" Of the patients admitted during the year, several have come to the asylum in restraints, which have of course always and immediately been removed. In no case has this removal been productive of any accident, or of any inconvenience or difficulty which the officers and attendants of a well-ordered asylum should not be expected to meet, and to overcome. Thirteen of the cases admitted were reported suicidal. The imposition of restraint in some of the cases alluded to appeared inexplicable; as the subjects of them were remarkable for their tranquillity.

" Two female patients among those who had been subjected to severe restraints before coming to the county asylum, had become insane in the puerperal state; and both began to recover almost as soon as admitted. One was an irritable patient, easily excited ; the other a delicate and timid woman, easily alarmed. These were among the few cases received at an early stage of the malady ; and both patients left the asylum within a few months after admission. (M. B. admitted December, 1844, and discharged March, 1845; and H. L. admitted February, 1845, and discharged March 28th.)

"Without making further allusion to the subject of restraint, I shall on this occasion merely observe that the sixth year, during which the great experiment of managing every kind of case without having recourse to it by day or by night, has been completed without the occurrence of any accident which restraint could have effectually prevented, and without the occurrence of any suicide; and that the non-restraint system appears to be becoming gradually adopted in the greater number of asylums, public and private."

FROM MY EIGHTH REPORT (1846).

" On the 21st day of September last, seven years were completed during which no strait-waistcoat, muff, leg-lock, handcuff, coercion-chair, or other means of mechanical restraint have been resorted to in the Hanwell Asylum, by night or by day. In those seven years, 1,100 cases have been admitted, and treated entirely on the non-restraint system; and the number of patients in the asylum has, during a great part of the same period, amounted to nearly 1,000.

" There are still some asylums in England, Ireland, and Scotland, in which such means of restraint are employed and defended; and travellers from various parts of the Continent, and from the United States of America, apparently prepossessed in favour of such ancient and forcible methods of control, continue to pay hasty visits to Hanwell, and to publish opinions condemnatory of the non-restraint system. In the annual reports of past years, when the experiment was but in an early stage of its progress, and when it was embarrassed by many difficulties, I refrained from engaging in any controversy on the subject; being satisfied that the results would furnish the best test of its being rational and judicious, as well as humane. If such results had not appeared, it would have been my duty to modify or abandon the system, as, in similar circumstances, it would have been my duty to alter or relinquish any other particular in the treatment of the patients. Now, after seven years' patient trial, during which the non-restraint system has been introduced into many other asylums, without the occurrence of any accident against which mechanical restraint would have afforded security, I do not think it desirable more particularly to notice the opinions of writers who have sometimes appeared to visit Hanwell more prepared to argue than disposed to observe; nor should I deem it necessary to refer to this part of the treatment, if it were not that I consider it still requisite to remind those who are most anxious to adopt it, that certain conditions are essential to its being successfully maintained.

" One of the first of these is, a properly constructed building, in which the patients enjoy the advantages of light and air, and a cheerful prospect, and ample space for exercise, and for classification, and means of occupation and recreation. The next is the constant and watchful superintendence of humane and intelligent officers, exercising full but considerate and just control over an efficient body of attendants. Other conditions are connected with such attention to the diet, clothing, lodging, and general cleanliness of the patients, as may exclude all avoidable sources of physical and mental uneasiness. Various employments, a certain extent of instruction, judicious religious attentions, and frequent opportunities of recreation, are indispensable and powerful auxiliaries. The whole treatment, management, and government of the patients and of the asylum, must, in short, be primarily adapted to the cure or improvement of infirm and disordered minds and bodies ; and as far removed, on the one hand, from the economy and organization of a workhouse, as, on the other, from the restrictions of a prison.

" In any public asylum constructed and conducted on these principles, and provided with proper resources against accidents incidental to all houses in which a number of insane persons are collected, the practicability and safety of the non-restraint system have now been satisfactorily proved by trials made in some of the largest of such institutions, and continued for several years. Every year in such asylums shows the possibility of removing more restrictions, and of dispensing with some of the precautions for which severe measures constituted the real necessity ; so that in every year the comfort and freedom of the patients admits of some further augmentation, and their condition becomes more assimilated to that of the sane, except in points for which their malady intrinsically disqualifies them; and for which an eventual remedy is sought by the indirect operation of a treatment calculated to relieve the feeble from responsibilities they are unequal to bear, from duties they are unable to perform, and all the unavoidable excitements of social life, which the morbidly irritable brain cannot endure.

" The wards of the Hànwell Asylum afford many illustrations of these principles. From some of them, the massive and immoveable tables and other furniture, once supposed to be necessary for safety, have been removed, and more convenient and moveable tables and seats of lighter construction put in their places; many of the window-guards have been found unnecessary; and various additional comforts, including coir-matting on the stone floor by the side of each bed, and a better kind of pillow, have been introduced into the sleeping rooms. The over-crowded state of the larger dormitories has been remedied by lessening the number of beds in them as far as practicable; whilst the admission of light and air has been greatly increased in those apartments by removing the earth or the walls which formerly obstructed the windows, so as to form gentle slopes covered with grass. A great addition to the winter comfort of many of the patients, and to the health of some of the older and feebler among them has been made by the formation of open fire-places in several of the day-rooms. Lavatories, or washing-rooms, have been added to many of the wards, and contribute much to the cleanliness and personal comfort of many of the patients. The substitution of cocoa for gruel, at breakfast, has given universal satisfaction; and the occasional substitution of a currant dumpling for soup, on the only soup-day in the week, has removed almost the only cause of discontent with the general dietary. Allowing white delf plates, and nickel forks, shaped like an ordinary dinner fork, to be used instead of the iron plates and very unsightly as well as more dangerous forks formerly used, has given an air of neatness to the dinner-table in several of the wards, which will, in all probability, be gradually extended to the rest. The tranquil and orderly patients have had the first benefit of some of these changes; and subsequently, the infirm, whose hands are often nearly helpless, and to whom the former forks, especially, were very inconvenient; but the other alterations have been more general. The extreme order with which the patients sit down to dinner, particularly on the male side of the asylum, and even in what are called the refractory wards, leaves no room for doubting that all the patients may in time participate in the benefit of every one of these improvements."

FROM MY ELEVENTH REPORT (1849).

" Ten years of the trial of a system of treatment
at the Hanwell asylum, from which all methods of
mechanical restraint have been strictly excluded,
were completed at the end of the month of September, 1849. Although it was deeply gratifying to
hear from the chairman of the additional asylum
for the county of Middlesex now erecting at Colney
Hatch, on the occasion of the foundation-stone
of the new building being laid in May last, by
H. R. H. the Prince Albert, that no mechanical
restraint would ever be introduced there, it is
discouraging to observe that such rude methods of
controlling the insane are yet practised and vindi-
cated in some of our largest public asylums, and to
know that they are carried to the extent of great
abuse in several private establishments. These
abuses, and the unnecessary and hurtful imposition
of restraints, are still defended on the plea that the
restraint of a strait-waistcoat is preferable to the
restraint of the hands of powerful attendants;
although it has been again and again explained
that the substitution of the attendants' hands, and
the selection of attendants merely on account of
their physical strength, has never formed any

part of the system of non-restraint as pursued at Hanwell.

" Permission to visit the asylum at Hanwell is so easily obtained that no real excuse exists for these continued, although unintentional, misrepresentations in medical reports and journals of recent date. Refraining, as it has been my rule to do, from controversy on these subjects, I would still urgently invite attention to the actual state of the asylum every day in the year, and every hour of the day. It seems impossible for any one possessing ordinary powers of observation and comparison, and an ordinary share of reason, not to find in its habitual condition the amplest justification of the system maintained there.

" I will only further simply state, that now, for ten entire years, no hand or foot has been fastened in this large asylum by day or by night, for the control of the violent or the despairing; that no instrument of mechanical restraint has been employed or even admitted into the wards for any reason whatever ; that no patient has been placed in a coercion-chair by day, or fastened to a bedstead at night; and that every patient, however excited or apparently unmanageable, arriving at the asylum in restraints, has been immediately set free and remained so from that time. I wish to overstate nothing ; but I am justified in adding, that the results, more and more seen in every successive year, have been increased tranquillity, diminished danger, and so salutary an influence over the recent and newly admitted, and most violent cases, as to make the spectacle of the more terrible forms of mania and melancholia a rare exception to the general order and cheerfulness of the establishment.

"I must add, for the satisfaction of those who have ever been led to suppose that severe medical means of restraint have been rendered necessary, and relied upon in the absence of restraints, that, among the substitutes for mechanical restraints, the temporary seclusion of patients — that salutary exclusion of causes of excitement from an already irritated brain, which has so unjustly been stigmatised as solitary imprisonment—is found to be but seldom necessary, except for a few hours, and as an actual remedy which the soundest principles of medicine would recognise in every disease of excitement. The douche-bath is never employed, in any case ; and the shower-bath is rarely resorted to, except for medical reasons ; whilst window-guards, dresses of very strong materials, strong blanket cases, and all the inventions required to limit the mischiefs to which many patients are prone, are only required in a proportion of cases very small in relation to the whole. But it ought never to be forgotten that the necessity for such resources must always depend on the character of the officers and attendants in an asylum. The great and only real substitute for restraint is invariable kindness. This feeling must animate every person employed, in every duty to be performed. Constant superintendence and care, constant forbearance and command of temper, and a never-failing attention to the comfort of the patients ; to their clothing, their food, their personal cleanliness, their occupations, their recreations ; these are but so many different ways in which such kindness shows itself; and these will be found to produce results beyond the general expectation of those who persevere in their application. Negligence on the part of the officers, and severity on the part of the attendants, will bring even the non-restraint system into disrepute, and create difficulties, and evils, and dangers against which bonds of leather and iron may, with apparent reasonableness, be represented as indispensable means of protection. In the wards of Hanwell, however, may still be pointed out some patients whom it was once considered unsafe to liberate from handcuffs or leg-locks ; who passed every day in the irksome confinement of a coercion-chair, and were every night secured by straps or chains ; and who have now been free for ten years, without evil consequences to others ; and with so much benefit to themselves, that their character seems to be entirely altered ; that they are seldom even secluded; and are even to be seen occasionally at the evening entertainments given to the patients, and already so often described.

" The whole of this subject occupied so much of my earlier reports (1839 to 1844) that, trusting such particular allusion to it as I have made on this particular occasion will be considered excusable, it is probable that I may seek no further opportunity of enforcing views which my experience continually confirms. For my own part in what has been undertaken, or in what has been accomplished, I trust I have never shown a desire to overstate it. I have always acknowledged myself indebted to Dr. Charlesworth and to Mr. Hill (of Lincoln) for the original suggestion of managing the insane without restraint. The magistrates of Middlesex gave me, ten years ago, the opportunity of attempting this on the greatest scale ; and they have honoured me, in all those years, with their steady support, in relation to the great principle of non-restraint. I owe much to the assistance of many able officers, who have devoted themselves to overcoming many incidental difficulties. Above all, I have never forgotten on what higher aid the success of all human attempts to accomplish good depends. My inward thought, in all the steps of the attempt which it has been my privilege to make, has still ever been, ' *Quia fuisti Adjutor meus !* ' "

In effecting all the alterations alluded to in the foregoing reports, I must again record the steady support of the committee of magistrates. With very few exceptions, they all liberally and courageously adopted the various suggestions made to them; and, without the particular zeal and perse-verance of some of their number, especially of Mr. Tulk, the chairman, and of Mr. Serjeant Adams, it is doubtful whether or not such great changes could ever have been effected; as, with the exception of the matron (Miss Powell, now Mrs. Bowden), the officers of the asylum at first regarded most of the innovations with various degrees of distrust. I had often, and more and more toward the close of my connection with the ordinary duties of Hanwell, to lament what seemed to me the imperfect views of the committee respecting the proper government, discipline, and subordi-nation required in an asylum; but I invariably found them animated by a humane consideration for the comfort of the patients, and always prompt to promote it in any manner pointed out to them, as well as by various methods which suggested themselves to their own minds.

Among the attempts which never, I think, received their general encouragement, were that of instructing the patients by means of schools; and that of imparting clinical instruction to medical pupils, so as more widely to diffuse the principles and practice which they sanctioned. Schools for the patients were twice instituted at Hanwell, and twice suppressed. On their second establishment, in 1847, the committee expressly stated that the schools were " not designed merely for instruction of patients in reading and writing, and similar matters, but for the awakening and improving the intellectual state of the imbecile and idiotic, and for the cultivation and gratification by instruction in natural history, geography, and general knowledge, of those patients who are already partially educated and instructed, and so as to excite, relieve, and recreate, as well as inform their minds." Such enlightened views could not be communicated to all the officers of the asylum; and the intentions of the committee, and the wishes of the medical officers and the chaplain, were frustrated. No attempt is now made to instruct the patients by these methods, always unfavourably regarded by those who estimate the mere work done by patients as of more importance than their mental improvement. But the systematic instruction which was given was found to be very useful to several patients, the cultivation of whose faculties had never received previous attention; and was certainly highly interesting and agreeable to others, in whom it revived knowledge long obscured in the struggle of life, or in the confusion of madness.

The chaplains successively attached to the asylum at the time the schools existed (the Rev. J. T. Burt, and the Rev. John May), not only approved but zealously favoured these efforts to instruct the ignorant, to assist the feeble-minded, and to add to the alleviations of the afflicted. They believed, as I did, that the schools consti- tuted a useful part of the system of treatment, and appeared to be impressed, as I was, with the instances witnessed at Hanwell, of patients learning to read and write with much satisfaction to them- selves, and the apparent sense of acquiring new faculties. Their progressive improvement, and the undeniable advancement of the mental character of some of them, including various favourable changes in their habits, were, indeed, too frequently noticed by me, when the schools were under the able and kind superintendence of Mr. and Miss Waite, to permit me to doubt that the institution of schools is a highly desirable part of the constitution of a public lunatic asylum.

With the suppression of the schools, the discon- tinuance of elementary lectures on subjects of natural history easy of comprehension was neces- sarily associated, and, indeed, every attempt to act on the remaining intellect of the patients. Together with these privations, many sources of happiness, of mental composure, and, as I believe, of means auxiliary to recovery, were also arbitrarily cut off. Such advantages were not, perhaps, of a nature to be estimated by the ordinary calculation of men of business; but the annual cost of a master and mistress, for advantages not to be so counted, of 150*l.* per annum, in an expenditure of 25,000*l.*, seemed an important retrenchment—for the old vice of economy was not extinct.

The steadiness with which the instruction of adult patients has been conducted for many years past in the asylum of the Bicêtre does honour to the French physicians, and to the governing autho- rities ; and we are doubtless much indebted to them for having set the example of extending the instruction, with judicious adaptations, to idiots and to imbecile children. It would be advantageous to many patients in the large asylums of England, and especially of those of Middlesex, where the patients, generally speaking, are most capable of improvement, if the members of the committees would pay some attention to what is effected, not only in Paris, but at the Earlswood asylum, near Reigate, and at Essex Hall, near Colchester. In these institutions, the results of the careful cultiva- tion of many intellects appearing at first of little promise have been successful beyond what the benevolent founders of those institutions dared to hope, or those who have not visited such institutions can believe.

Committees of management, composed as those of the large asylums near London are, may be excused if, contemplating the comforts they have provided for the pauper lunatic, they consider their performance complete. But the medical officers cannot fall into such error. They know, and ought to be influenced by their knowledge of, what is attempted and what is accomplished in other countries, as in France and in Germany, where not only the insane· but the imbecile and idiotic are made the objects of careful, ingenious, various, and yet systematic education. Within an easy journey, they may now study the application of similar attention extended to children of all degrees of limited capacity in our own country; and they should be the last to give countenance to the depreciation of such attempts by those who have not time, or inclination, or patience, to examine and consider them, and thus truly to estimate their results. And, if their hope now and then fails them, they should call to mind the exertions of the American physician and philanthropist, Dr. Howe, whose earnest and courageous efforts in the case of Laura Bridgman awakened into exercise, in one deaf, and blind, and dumb, all the faculties of a living soul.

In neglecting to open the wards of Hanwell and

Colney Hatch to students of medicine, the committees of those asylums also assuredly neglect a kind of duty to the public. They could not, however, conveniently do so without a larger medical staff, and the means of keeping fuller records of the numerous cases than are compatible with the laborious duties already thrown on the medical officers. It is still to be hoped that this subject will obtain due attention; and that the early treatment of insane persons, in all classes of life, will not always continue, as it now is, to be of necessity entrusted to those who, although competently educated in medicine and surgery, and their auxiliary sciences, have never had opportunities of becoming practically acquainted with disorders particularly manifesting themselves in mental disorder. In all asylums the statistical registers show that the recoveries, in the recent cases admitted, are in the first year numerous; that in the second year from the commencement of the malady they are much fewer; and that in the third and subsequent years they become rare. Not only in pauper practice, but in practice generally, the treatment of the insane is conducted, often for the first two or three months, always for the first two or three weeks, by medical men engaged and skilful in general practice, but unpractised in these severe forms of cerebral disorder, and disconcerted and alarmed by their occurrence among their patients. Anxious to acquire some insight into such maladies, which they observe often to run on to hopeless forms of insanity, and not unfrequently to be followed by unexpected and fatal results, they find it still scarcely possible to obtain such admission to the wards of asylums as would give them the experience required to remove their often recurring anxieties.

These circumstances make it highly important, in regard to the pauper lunatics, that the medical officers of district unions, to whom all the cases of insanity occurring among the poor of the district are necessarily at first confided, should be better prepared than it is possible for them now to be to recognise the different forms of mental malady, and well acquainted with the treatment found to be most successful in asylums. In such institutions, according to modern experience, one-half, perhaps two-thirds, of the recent cases recover: whilst not one-third, perhaps not one-tenth, of those recover who are injudiciously treated on the first appearance of the malady. To increase the facilities of medical students, and even of medical men engaged in practice, of acquiring the knowledge necessary for the proper management of cases of insanity is an object worthy of the serious consideration of the council of the University of London; and of all the governing bodies of medical schools. The East India Company have already recognised these views; and have set an example worthy of being followed.

In the Parisian asylums, a larger staff of medical officers has enabled the directors to make those institutions more subservient to study and science than those of London. Pinel was, I believe, the first to give clinical lessons; Dr. Falret alludes to lectures of this character given in 1814*; Esquirol, the successor of Pinel, received pupils and delivered lectures at the Salpêtrière during the nine years from 1817 to 1826. Many of those who had enjoyed the advantage of this instruction became afterward the superintendents of provincial asylums, and diffused throughout the country the enlightened views of the great teachers of the capital. Dr. Ferrus, now inspector-general of asylums in France, attracted many pupils by his able lectures at the Bicêtre, from 1832 to 1839: Dr. Leuret afterward gave lectures also at the Bicêtre. In 1843, after much consideration had been given to various objections made to the admission of pupils into lunatic asylums, the council of that asylum authorised Dr. Falret and Dr. Baillarger to continue a course of teaching which they had commenced, Dr. Falret in that year, and Dr. Leuret in 1841. Clinical lessons appear to have been given in many of the German asylums, since

* De L'Enseignement Clinique des Maladies Mentales. Paris, 1850, p. 15.

Dr. Horn began the practice at Berlin, and Dr. Müller at Wurtzburg. Autenrieth, Joseph Frank, and Nasse, were among the distinguished German physicians who gave this kind of instruction.

Very little activity has yet been shown as regards such instruction in England. The clinical teaching at Bethlem Hospital, commenced by Sir Alexander Morison, was from some cause or other of very limited use to students; and although now countenanced and even enforced by the governors of that institution, imposes a heavy duty on Dr. Hood, the physician, already overburdened with duties. At St. Luke's, regular courses of lectures have at length been instituted by Dr. A. Sutherland and Dr. H. Monro. At Hanwell, clinical teaching was commenced in 1842. It appeared to me that then only could the proper study of insanity begin; the removal of restraints, and of all violent and irritating methods of control, then first permitting the student to contemplate disorders of the mind in their simplicity, and no longer modified by exasperating treatment. Patients could then be presented to their observation as subjects of study and reflection, and not as criminals; and regarded as persons to be cured of illness, or relieved from distress, and not as beings to be tortured by confinement of the limbs, or mortified by punishments. Scenes of general confusion and agitation, opposed to the possibility of study, had become rare; the wards were tranquil, the patients were cheerful; and the visits of the pupils were looked forward to with interest. The actual state of the minds of the insane was in most cases easily displayed to the learner, without the least distress to the patient; and the effects of treatment were readily appreciated. Among the early pupils, some have since had opportunities of putting in practice what they learned at Hanwell; and in no instance have I known them abandon the system with which they there became acquainted. But the clinical instruction at Hanwell was impeded by many obstacles. The lecturer's means of commanding the assistance he required were limited and uncertain; and after some interruptions, principally arising from this cause, all attempts at clinical teaching have been given up. In the additional asylum for Middlesex, at Colney Hatch, no attempt of the kind has been made: and although the Directors of the East India Company have required, since the beginning of 1852, that the assistant-surgeons in their service shall have had practical instruction in an asylum for the treatment of the insane, for at least three months, the opportunity of doing so in either of the large establishments for the county of Middlesex, where such instruction would be so valuable, and so eagerly sought, has not yet been afforded.

A serious error, existing especially in some of

the large asylums near London, lies at the root of
all these defects. To keep the number of medical
officers as small as possible, and to give them
the smallest possible degree of authority, seems to
be much the aim of the governing bodies; who
appear, indeed, scarcely to associate the idea of
a medical staff with anything but the administration
of physic. Their guides and counsellors in asylum
matters are never selected from the physicians.
They are never seen in the wards with their
medical officers, whose influence on the patients
they seem to have no curiosity about. Of all parts
of committee business, that which is productive of
the most impatience is the medical part; and the
medical suggestions are usually received with small
respect. Such was too often the case, even at
Hanwell, after the first enthusiasm for the new
method of treatment had passed away; and proposi-
tions to increase the medical service of the house,
and to make it more effective, by the aid of clinical
pupils, which would have involved scarcely any
expense, were rejected as not worth discussing.
The constitution of the French asylums appears
to be better; at least the council of the French
hospitals for the insane show, by their medical
appointments, that they do not consider one
physician, or even two physicians, whatever their
zeal and devotedness to their duties, able to give
all the attention that is required from them to

1,500 or even to 800 insane patients. At the Salpêtrière there are three physicians and two assistant-physicians; the number of patients being about 1,300: and at the Bicêtre two physicians and two assistant-physicians, for 800 patients: and among these physicians and assistants there is not one who has not already attained eminence in the profession, or who is not more or less known by his writings. The influence of a medical staff so efficient, both in number and reputation, is unquestionable; and in all the regulations of those asylums it is observable that the opinions of the medical officers are always respectfully considered.

In the asylum of Illenau, in Germany, there are only 450 patients, many of whom are of the poorer class; but there are four medical officers attached to it, under Dr. Roller, who is the physician in chief. At the Siegburgh institution there are three medical officers, and not more than 200 patients. Medical duties and medical influences are evidently looked upon as more important than they appear to be in the large establishments for the insane paupers of Middlesex and Surrey, or at Bethlem and St. Luke's. It is very probable that if the members of the committees of these large institutions knew the nature of the incessant duties of their medical officers, they would not disregard these considerations; and, certainly, if the public could really estimate the consequences of the present inadequate number of medical officers in relation to the duties which at least ought to be performed in asylums, an augmentation would be insisted upon. With the various interruptions to which they are liable, it is quite evident that two medical officers cannot sufficiently superintend 1,000 patients; that they cannot even visit the wards sufficiently often without exhaustion; and consequently cannot exercise due superintendence over the attendants; that on numerous occasions, important attentions must be omitted, and important circumstances overlooked; and that many special moral appliances must be neglected, with serious consequences to the patients, not the less real because they are unrecorded. The want of a medical chief in these great buildings—to which Bethlem is the only exception—is also a great evil; for which the fancied efficiency of committees and sub-committees affords no kind of compensation. It implies a want of any uniform plan, and of all effective co-operation among the officers. It enables them all in turn to obtain the sanction of some of the committee to something at variance with the system professed to be maintained; and it also enables the committee to control every officer in turn by the pernicious system of antagonism. Until these defects attract attention, no system, however excellent, will rest, in any asylum, on a secure foundation. There is no principle which seems more self-evident than that, in asylums for the insane, nothing should be done without the approbation of the chief physician, or of the medical officers. Every change in the rules, and every alteration in the building, affects the patients favourably or unfavourably; and of the manner in which they will be affected the medical men are the most competent judges. The many alterations made in asylums at variance with all good principles, are to be explained by their being resolved upon without medical sanction, or in contemptuous disregard of it. The size of asylums has increased, and is increasing to a most objectionable extent; so that desperate measures are resorted to, and cases of poor paralysed lunatics begin to be excluded from the kind care of such institutions, or delivered back to the workhouses. By such means money is saved, and the institutions appear less expensive; but also become less conducive to the comfort and recovery of the patients. As the buildings extend, the duties of the officers increase, and neglects multiply. And as regards the economical discovery that the paralytics may be consigned to workhouse-treatment, it may certainly have the effect of causing them to be for a shorter time burthensome to the public, or to the county; but no medical man can approve of such an arrangement, which is as inconsistent with the proper scope of the art of healing as it is with common humanity.

Without a very efficient superintendence, chiefly to be exercised by the medical officers, or rather by a chief medical officer, the mere absence of mechanical restraint may constitute no sufficient security against the neglect or even the actual ill-treatment of insane persons in a large asylum. The medical officers of asylums who consider such watchful superintendence not properly comprised in their duties, have formed a very inadequate conception of their duties. Committees content to allow a treasurer, a steward, or a head attendant, or a matron and her assistants, to be relied upon for such superintendence, unknowingly neglect a great duty to the insane whom they have undertaken to protect. Under an indolent or careless medical officer, no real security can be afforded even against gross cruelty. Seclusion or the shower-bath may be so abused as to be converted into punishments; the old and wicked custom of depriving the patients of food when they have been refractory, may be revived; the attendants may habitually practise various forms of intimidation; may make the patients suffer various privations; and, when provoked, may resort to the plan of half strangling them, in order to overcome resistance, or to secure obedience in some particular which ought, perhaps, at least to be postponed, or even is not properly insisted upon at all. Practices of this kind have been proved to be common in some asylums; and they may long escape detection where there is no active medical head. With proper superintendence, they would be almost impossible.

PART V.

GRADUAL ADOPTION OF THE NON-RESTRAINT SYSTEM IN THE LARGE ASYLUMS OF ENGLAND, AFTER 1839.

As soon as the new system of treatment had been fairly tried at Hanwell, it began to be adopted by the superintendents of several English asylums, approaching nearest to Hanwell in size. Success followed everywhere. It was invariably found that when there was a determination to manage all cases of insanity without resorting to the employment of mechanical coercion, it was practicable, and safe, and advantageous to do so. What first appeared exceptions were by degrees heard of no more, and apparent failures were seen to be the result of some incompleteness in the application of the new system. In whatever asylum it found a favourable consideration, its acceptance was a sure consequence, and no instance of subsequent abandonment of it occurred. Neither the successive superintendents who adopted it, nor myself, ventured to say, with **Mr. Gardiner Hill**, that a case might not possibly occur in which the rule of non-restraint must be departed from; but they and I equally well knew, or gradually learned, that in a well constructed and well governed asylum, with proper attendants, such a concession need scarcely be made. The experience of the years which have passed over since the experiment began, has fully confirmed this confidence.

The officers of the asylums at Hanwell and Colney Hatch must have seen so many instances of the most violent patients soon restored to calmness, and of the most desperately suicidal preserved from often-recurring paroxysms of dangerous tendency, and of paralytic and helpless patients kept clean and comfortable, without the resort, in any case, to a coercion-chair, a strait-waistcoat, a handcuff, a muff, a leg-lock, a chain or strap, or any device by which the movements of the patient were impeded, and his temper needlessly fretted, that I have no doubt a very large volume of such cases might be compiled from those two asylums alone.

To those who have learned to care for the insane, the establishment, within the last few years, of many admirable county asylums has been an event of a very interesting kind, because such institutions have in hundreds of instances sheltered the poorer lunatic from indescribable miseries. I have no doubt that all of these new institutions could furnish illustrations of patients brought to them in a state approaching death, and yet who revived, and were preserved, and restored to mental and bodily health. The diminution of suffering thus occasioned is among the most gratifying results of this age, in which, almost for the first time since the formation of human societies, the higher and richer classes have turned their attention to the condition of the daily state of the poor and lowly, to their comfortless homes and hourly privations, and have carried the principle of mercy into all the abodes of obscure want and affliction.

Success has still been commensurate to these provisions for the insane, and, to a certain extent, even in cases where previous years of neglect have almost effaced all human characteristics. In Dr. Hitchman's first report of the Derbyshire asylum (1853) we read of a male patient brought to that institution naked, except that around the pelvis there were some remains of a dress: his hands were tightly bound. "He roared hideously as he was being conveyed to the wards." The patient was of large size and formidable aspect; but he appeared to be unable to retain the erect posture without support. He resisted all attempts to clothe him, and he seemed unacquainted with the use of a bedstead. "He whined after the manner of a dog that has lost its home;" that home appearing to have been, for more than thirty years, a mere outhouse. He seemed to dread everybody, and he was lost to all sense of decency. " He is guided," says Dr. Hitchman's description of him on admission, " by the lowest instincts only; and his whole appearance and manner, his fears, his whines, his peculiar skulking from observation, his bent gait, his straight hair, large lips, and gigantic forearm, painfully remind one of the more sluggish of the anthropoid apes, and tell but too plainly to what sad depths the human being can sink, under the combined influence of neglect and disease."

It is interesting to know what impression could possibly be made on such a case as this, even in an asylum comprehending every possible advantage. Fifteen months after his admission, Dr. Hitchman was able to say of him :—" He now walks about the galleries properly clothed, smiles when he is approached, puts out his hand in a friendly manner towards those he recognises, sits regularly at meals, is shaved at appointed times, carries himself nearly erect, and looks as if he belonged to the children of men."

In the above case, there appears to have been no violence to contend with ; but another patient, admitted into the same asylum from a workhouse, had been shouting " Murder!" all night, at the top of his voice, so as to alarm the neighbourhood. He had knocked down one attendant, and appeared to " have the strength of an elephant." " One of three men who brought him," says Dr. Hitchman, " stated that his finger had been severely crushed by the patient, who pinioned him between the door and its post, and kept him there for more than an hour. If ever restraint was needed, it was with this man. He is six feet high, very muscular, and with a wrist which few persons can span. He was brought to the asylum firmly pinioned by ropes and handbolts, and his arms were severely bruised from this cause. In a few minutes all the manacles were removed; he has had the perfect use of every limb since he has been in the asylum, and has been fully controlled by moral means alone."

Thirty suicidal cases were admitted at Derby in about eighteen months. In some of them desperate attempts had been made at self-destruction. Some required watching day and night; but no restraint was resorted to, and no suicide occurred.

These are, we may now say, the constant results of the non-restraint system, fully carried out by those who understand it, and who can command the various resources required when fastening the limbs is no longer relied upon; and who are resolved that no difficulties shall impel them to acts inconsistent with that goodwill and confidence of the patients towards them which impart to a superintendent almost miraculous influence and power. If the physician is benevolent and enlightened, if his officers are faithful and trustworthy, and he has proper authority over them and the attendants, such a task becomes at length easy in the performance, and even a lunatic asylum becomes the abode of comfort and peace.

For several years the progress of this method in England generally remained very slow; and the explanation of this was the same, I believe, as is that of the hostility to it which still exists on the part of the German and French physicians. Physicians and superintendents of asylums wrote against it; reasoned against it; expressed themselves angrily against it; but scarcely any of them devoted any time to observing it. A few reflecting men were happily found who did devote more than an hour or two, or than even a day or two, to watching the results of non-restraint. One of these was Mr. Gaskell, now a Commissioner in Lunacy; and it is well known that he adopted the system, and carried it out with singular ability and success in the large asylum of Lancaster, where he had to control many patients whose provincial character was proverbially rough and brutal. There, as at Hanwell, walls were lowered, iron bars removed, the means of exercise and recreation increased; so as to introduce the whole system of non-restraint into an asylum then containing 600 patients. Mr. Gaskell was soon able to report that there were several among them who had become active and cleanly, and cheerful, and contented, who had formerly been in the strictest mechanical restraint, and had then been in a state in every respect the reverse.

Another careful observer was the late Dr. Anderson, who visited Hanwell several times on his appointment as superintendent of the lunatic asylum attached to the Naval Hospital at Haslar. Previous to his taking the charge of the patients there, then about 120 in number, including twenty or thirty naval officers, some of the patients were constantly in restraints, being accounted incurably dangerous. One of them was always in handcuffs; but he had learned to put his hands into all of his several pockets, and to use them so freely that the protection was merely imaginary, and the restraint merely unnecessarily troublesome and vexatious. Eighteen patients slept in iron handcuffs, chained to their beds; their feet also being fastened. There were, however, no restraint chairs in the building. To all the windows there were heavy iron bars. The patients were not entrusted with knives and forks. In the airing courts there were many refreshing plots of grass, but the patients were not allowed to walk on them. There were no shrubberies. The view of the sea, of Portsmouth harbour, and of the Isle of Wight, was shut out by very high walls. Dr. Anderson had not been long there before everything underwent a favourable change. Restraints were entirely abolished; iron bars disappeared; the boundary walls were lowered; the patients were allowed to walk upon the grass; summer - houses were built, and pleasant seats provided commanding a view of the sea, and the cheerful scenes most congenial to the inmates; knives and forks were brought into use; and the whole of this noble asylum assumed an air of tranquil comfort. The patients soon had a large boat provided for them, in which their good physician did not hesitate to trust himself with parties of them, in fishing excursions. In the first of these little voyages a patient, whose voice had not been heard for years, was so delighted with his success that he counted his fish aloud. These changes were all effected without accident or inconvenience. The patients reputed to be dangerous had under this new management proved to be trustworthy; and some of them became industriously occupied. Throughout Dr. Anderson's attempt he was steadily supported and countenanced by Sir William Burnett, then at the head of the medical department of the navy. Our gallant soldiers are not yet provided with a similar asylum for the reception of the insane, which is much to be regretted; but the deficiency will doubtless soon be supplied.

I record with pleasure, also, the instance of Dr. Hutcheson, then superintendent of the Glasgow asylum, who devoted several visits to making himself acquainted with the system pursued at Hanwell, and subsequently carried it out so successfully, that when the new asylum was built at Gartnavel, near Glasgow, an inscription on the foundation-stone recorded that into that institution mechanical restraint was never to be introduced. This was among the Scotch, who were confidently predicated to be ungovernable by any but strong methods.

Dr. Davey was for some time (from 1840 to 1844) one of the medical officers at Hanwell ; and he subsequently practised the non-restraint system with signal success among the insane in Ceylon, even in the miserable places allotted to them by the local government in that colony, in 1844. Since that time he has had an opportunity of introducing the same system on the female side of the asylum at Colney Hatch ; whilst Dr. Hood pursued it on the male side. It should be remembered that these two physicians undertook the whole medical responsibility of this new asylum, large enough for the reception of 1,200 patients, without thinking it necessary to have a single strait-waistcoat or any instrument of restraint in the whole building. Dr. Hood has more recently established the same system at Bethlem Hospital ; formerly the fastness of every form and variety of exceptionable treatment.

Dr. Nesbitt succeeded Dr. Davey at Hanwell, and has since fully maintained the system at

Northampton. Dr. Hitchman succeeded Dr. Nesbitt, and under his superintendence there is not a better governed asylum in England than that of Derbyshire, over which he now presides. To the able, zealous, and friendly co-operation of these estimable men, when they were officers at Hanwell, it is a sincere gratification to me to refer. Their kindness and skill helped to overcome many difficulties, and to alleviate many cares.

I believe I may add that Dr. Hitch and Dr. Williams of Gloucestershire, Dr. Bucknill of Devonshire, Dr. Thurnam of Wiltshire, Dr. Diamond of Surrey, Dr. Parsey of Warwickshire, and other superintendents of large county asylums, were in some degree influenced by their acquaintance with Hanwell in resolving to act on the non-restraint system in their respective institutions. It is also to be observed that whilst the opponents of the non-restraint system have always been non-resident officers, the great measure of the abolition of restraints was only at first ventured upon by resident officers, whose constant observation gave them full assurance that it was safe.

For six or seven years clinical lectures were given at the Hanwell asylum. Every part of the asylum, and every patient, was shown to the pupils; and every thing was explained. I know that several of these gentlemen have since had opportunities of acting on the principles they learnt, and the convictions they received there; and that in no instance either they, or any physicians who, after studying the details of the non-restraint system, and then giving it a fair trial, have turned round, abandoned it, and resorted again to the miserable methods formerly relied upon.

The Commissioners in Lunacy, who were at first disposed to regard the new system with some disfavour, still carefully observed its progress and its results; and when they became convinced that it was really deserving of encouragement, promoted its progress by every means that they possessed; taking the utmost pains, in all their visitations, to abolish all that was objectionable in the old institutions, both public and private, and urging with unceasing earnestness, in their reports, the adoption of every improvement. At length, in their Eighth Report, published in 1854, they embodied an infinite number of details illustrative of the actual condition of all the asylums of England and Wales, as regarded the employment or disuse of restraints. The information widely diffused over the world by this official document, and the opinions expressed in it by the Commissioners themselves, must have been most extensively beneficial. It contained, especially, the replies made to the inquiries of the Commissioners by the superintendents of public and county asylums, the perusal of which, rather curiously contrasted with the replies sent from several of the private asylums, afforded great satisfaction to all interested in the abandonment of mechanical restraints.   The information thus obtained, in addition to that gathered from other sources, appeared to show that in about twenty-seven public or county asylums, in England and Wales, out of about thirty, mechanical restraints had then become wholly abolished, these asylums containing, altogether, about 10,000 patients.   In nine out of fourteen institutions for the insane called hospitals it also appeared that restraints were no longer resorted to ; these including Bethlem Hospital and St. Luke's ; and the total number of insane patients in the hospitals exceeding nine hundred.   In some of the hospitals not included in this statement, and especially in the York Retreat, containing one hundred patients, restraints were at that time so very rarely resorted to as to be almost wholly unused.

To the statements of the superintendents of asylums contained in this important report, all who desire to obtain a correct knowledge of the manner in which the non-restraint system has been found to act in the larger institutions, under the careful watching of prudent physicians, and of the improvements that invariably accompany its introduction, both as regards the patients and the attendants, may be confidently referred.   Such kind of information is now to be obtained from nearly every annual report published by the super-intendents of asylums. Dr. Bucknill has conferred no small service on the profession by his able analysis of the most recent of these, in the 17th number of the Asylum Journal, so ably conducted by him. He notices the interesting fact, that when the Eighth Report of the Commissioners was published, there were at least three county asylums to which the proprietors might point as giving countenance to the employment of mechanical restraint; and that the number is now (1856) reduced to one. Dr. Bucknill believes that there will soon be not one exception; and if the asylum for the North Riding of York now constitutes such an exception, we have the strongest confirmation of Dr. Bucknill's hope in its admirable general management, and in the cordial interest taken by Mr. Hill, the superintendent, in the general happiness of the patients under his charge; and his promotion among them of those agricultural occupations by which the asylum is enabled to supply a certain quantity of vegetables and fruit to the dealers from York, whose resort to the asylum in the early mornings of summer for this purpose, imparts cheerfulness and animation to many of its inmates.

The gradual advance of the new system has perhaps been marked by no circumstance more striking than by that of the opening of at least

ten English county asylums, of considerable size,
within the last few years, without any preparation
being considered necessary or desirable, in any
one of them, for any application of mechanical
restraints.   These asylums have been erected to
receive, altogether, about 4,000 patients; patients
of all descriptions—the violent, the melancholic,
and those rendered nearly intractable by long
misery.   It is among the glories of medical philosophy, which no false splendour enhances, and
which therefore attracts little popular regard,
that the physicians selected to govern these new
institutions undertook to do so by moral and
intellectual means alone.   So much more confident
were they, indeed, of the efficacy of these means
than of the effects of the old measures of force,
that they did not even require the windows of their
asylums to be guarded; and scarcely demanded
strong dresses, and the other substitutes for
restraints, which had become in every successive
year less required at Hanwell, and were found
to be scarcely required at all in the more
modern asylums in which restraints had never
been known.

The statements and sentiments contained, indeed,
in every report now issued from the English county
asylums, become, in every year, more uniformly
gratifying.   In the latest report of the Kent
asylum, Dr. Huxley, who has appeared reluctant

to abandon the defence of the occasional employ
ment of restraint, says:—"It is with no little
satisfaction that I find myself able to report the
fact of there having been no instance of mechanical
restraint throughout the year. This variation in
practice," he adds, "is not due to any change of
opinion, but simply to the non-occurrence of a case,
or of a condition, in which I believe restraining to
be necessary." This belief will, it is to be hoped,
be confirmed by every succeeding year; for, as Dr.
Bucknill observes in the article already referred to,
"it is a very remarkable fact, that not a single
report published during the year (1855) contains
the slightest or most indirect defence of the old
methods." In the first report of the Essex asylum,
containing 300 patients, Dr. Campbell, speaking
of the old system of coercion having now generally
been changed for one of freedom, says:—"This is
the principle according to which this asylum is
conducted; which, from its admirable construction
and general arrangements, I am enabled to carry
out to the full extent. Four hundred and thirty-
nine cases have been admitted; in no case has
mechanical restraint been resorted to, and no means
for such coercion exist in the establishment. It is
impossible to estimate too highly the beneficial
consequences of the non-restraint system when
aided by cleanliness, wholesome food, and employment or exercise in the open air; and a stronger

proof of its advantages cannot be adduced than
the feelings which were evinced by two of those
patients who had the misfortune of a second attack,
and returned to the asylum.   No horror was
exhibited at the prospect of a further period of
confinement; no dread of fetters; on the con-
trary, they seemed to return as if to a home
which they considered was happily prepared for
them."

The testimony of Dr. Palmer of the Lincolnshire
county asylum, containing 250 patients (second
report, 1855), and opened without the provision of
a single instrument of coercion, is of a like kind.
" It may be," says Dr. Palmer, " as some assert,
that time is still required to test this question
(non-restraint) fully ; and that a large number of
fresh cases must yet pass under treatment before
the total abolition of instrumental restraint can
be established as a principle ; but so far as the
experience of the superintendent of this asylum
goes, he is convinced that no more pernicious
agents were ever introduced into institutions for
the insane than mechanical contrivances to check
the disorderly outbursts of maniacal excitement,
or to antagonize the suicidal impulses of melancholy.
Whatever the effects of such rude means may be
on some rare and exceptional cases—whether
productive of injury or otherwise—he has no doubt
that their effects on the patients generally are to

excite perversity and resistance to moral control, and on the attendants, to inculcate a reliance on coercive measures rather than on those of a guiding and directing character. None of the presumed exceptional cases have as yet appeared in this asylum; nor has any instrument of restraint ever been within its walls, save to call for the pleasing duty of immediately removing it from the person of some newly arrived patient, and sending it away."

Dr. Sherlock, also, in the second report of the Worcester asylum, where there are more than 200 patients, observes that the asylum is conducted on the non-restraint system, and that no means of controlling a patient by restraints exist in the house.

To read of such views and practice among the superintendents of the new asylums is most satisfactory. In no institutions can the real difficulties of dispensing with mechanical coercion be more strongly felt than in large county asylums, thrown open all at once to a crowd of lunatics brought from private asylums, or from workhouses, or from the outhouses, and cells, and dens in which they have been previously kept. Yet no evidence is stronger or more decisive in favour of non-restraint than that given by the officers of the new asylums where all the appliances of coercion are unknown. It is, however, not to be forgotten, but to be gratefully acknowledged, that the committees of the

new provincial asylums, consisting generally of
gentlemen of station and education in their respective counties, greatly facilitate, by their liberal
views and the confidence they place in the superintending officer or physician, the maintenance of a
good system of treatment. Their reports manifest
a close attention to all the matters essential to a
good asylum. The situation, the aspect, the
character of the building, the supply of water, the
means of drainage, and of warming and ventilating
the galleries and rooms, and the promotion of
external cheerfulness of appearance by the formation of plantations and gardens, are objects
repeatedly dwelt upon and shown to be carefully
considered, as well as all the details of the interior,
concerning which it is in most of the provincial
asylums customary to consult the physician, whose
opinion as regards many of them is of greater
importance than the abstract views of architects.

In the older asylums, the medical officers
enjoyed few of these advantages, and the difficulty
of establishing an unexceptionable system of treatment in such buildings has only yielded to the
energy of physicians who would not regard difficulty
as a perpetual excuse for defects. No medical
officer should despair of succeeding in the attempt
to carry out the non-restraint system in any asylum
who has made himself acquainted with the obstacles
that were either to be overcome or unheeded in the

great hospital of Bethlem, by Dr. Hood, or that of St. Luke's, by Dr. Sutherland and Dr. Henry Monro, assisted by Dr. Arlidge, then the resident medical officer. Long established customs, based on long established prejudices, were to be overcome; numerous patients, above the class of paupers, and less obedient than paupers, were to be controlled and managed safely in buildings ill adapted to modern views, and having very limited grounds or other means for the diversion of the minds of the patients. Within the last few years the entire character of these institutions has been changed, and restraints are now banished from both of them, although the faults of construction, situation, and want of space, are in both irremediable. An asylum is still wanting near London for the reception of patients of the educated classes in indigent circumstances, and those of the middle classes generally; an asylum affording all the auxiliary advantages enjoyed in the county asylums by the pauper lunatic, and at the Northampton, Stafford, and Manchester asylums for those in question. Neither Bethlem nor St. Luke's can fully supply this deficiency, not from any incongruity of such an application of their funds with the constitution of those asylums, nor from any existing defects in the medical system pursued, but from the character of those buildings, and their situation.

Many years ago (in 1841) Mr. Wilkes, now a

Commissioner in Lunacy, showed the practicability of gradually dispensing with the use of restraints in the old asylum at Stafford, where, when he first took charge of it, he found " the leather muff and wrist-straps, iron handcuffs, long leather sleeves, hobbles for the legs, the restraint chair, and various devices specially adapted to the propensities and habits of the patients, freely employed both by day and night." Concerning these arrangements Mr. Wilkes observes:—" The evil of this system was not simply confined to the coercion of the patients, but the principle pervaded the whole establishment, and the high windows, in many instances protected by iron guards or wire-work, the numerous staples in the walls of the galleries and rooms for confining patients to their seats, and the strongly guarded fireplaces, gave a gloomy, prison-like aspect to the interior of the building, which was perpetuated externally by the cheerless high-walled airing courts, destitute of either trees or flowers." By cautious degrees all these arrangements were changed, and with a marked improvement in the character of the patients. With the removal of restraints, and the conversion of the gloomy airing courts into pleasant gardens, the patients became less troublesome and destructive by day, and less noisy and restless by night, and accidents of all kinds became less frequent. After about fourteen years' experience, during which upwards of fifteen hundred patients had been received into the Stafford asylum, Mr. Wilkes concluded his report for 1854 by stating that his opinion had been daily trengthened and confirmed that, as a general rule, " mechanical restraint employed in the treatment of the insane is both unnecessary and injurious."

One of the latest instances of signal amelioration in the state of an establishment for the insane has been presented by the asylum for the county of Bedford, containing about three hundred patients. A few years ago (1851) the committee were only able to express their pleasure that the amount of restraint used in the asylum had become greatly diminished ; but the medical officers at that time continued to be the advocates of what they called " mild restraint." In 1854, Mr. Denne, from the Hanwell asylum, was appointed resident superintendent ; and in his first report he was enabled to say that, notwithstanding many difficulties, and the general misconstruction of the building, he had wholly abolished mechanical restraint, that the patients had expressed themselves grateful for the change, and that, among other results, the quantity of clothing destroyed had become " immeasurably less." The banishment of restraints had been accompanied by an improved diet, an additional quantity of land for cultivation, improved clothing, and all the constituent parts of the non-restraint system compatible with the old building, which is about to be replaced by a new one, constructed according to the more enlightened ideas of modern times.

I refer again with satisfaction to the Derbyshire asylum, as it was one of the first erected in England with every advantage of experience on the part of the architect, Mr. Duesbury, of the things actually required in a large residence for the insane. It is unnecessary to say that under the direction of Dr. Hitchman, it became, and continues to be, an illustration of all that is liberal in management, and skilful and humane in treatment. No physician in this country seems to have paid earlier attention to the real results of abolishing mechanical restraints; and in his report, dated January 1855, he thus expressed himself:—" Never having hazarded any abstract speculations upon the subject, or indulged in theories as to what may or may not occur, your physician will, as heretofore, content himself with being simply the historian of his own experience. That experience commenced several years before the great experiment of non-restraint was tried at Hanwell, and embraced, therefore, the usual routine of strait-waistcoats, and all the paraphernalia of mechanical control; but he can most conscientiously aver, that not a single patient (in upwards of 2,000) has, during the past ten years, been restrained while under his observation. Many patients have been

under restraint at the period of their admission;
and such restraint was deemed by other medical
men to be urgently required. The following are
among such cases admitted into the asylum during
the past year. The facts within inverted commas
are derived from the certificates upon which the
patients were admitted. J. A., brought in chains.
' Has threatened to murder T. B. and T. E. with a
knife; has been in a state of great excitement for
four days, offering to fight.' G. H. and W. D. were
brought in restraints from an institution in which
restraints are professedly employed : they were very
violent. 'G. H. is now suffering from an attack of
acute mania, characterised by continued violence
and excitement, rendering it dangerous for any one
to approach him. His conversation is rapid and
full of delusions ; he shouts words without meaning,
as Punch Junior. He is at present under personal
restraint, having threatened violence to attendants
and destroyed bedding. R. H., attendant on the
insane, says, I saw G. H. before he was admitted—
it took several men to secure him—he threatened
to let out the entrails of several persons, and to
kill the first man he came to. Since his admission
he has refused his food ; has been in an excited
state, and threatened to knock a man's head off.
R. H. says W. D. frequently strikes the patients.
His conversation is full of debauchery ; he is
intolerable when the fits come on. Yesterday he

smashed with one of the fire-irons the sashes of
the window, and ten panes of glass; he threatens
to kill me, and ran after me with a poker; says he
will rip his own entrails clear out; considers himself
one of the best fellows in existence.' These cases,"
says Dr. Hitchman, "might be multiplied: they
were most powerful men, and in states of violent
excitement. One of them was much bruised. The
verbal statements made by those who brought them
were even stronger than the written account; yet,
in obedience to a principle which has hitherto been
unfailing, they were liberated immediately, and
never restrained again. One, who was a butcher
by trade, slaughtered a pig for the institution
within a fortnight after his chains were removed;
and from that time was employed daily in useful
occupations until he was discharged—cured. A
second has also returned home cured. The third
is an epileptic, and will probably remain with us as
long as he lives."

These instances seem fully to justify Dr. Hitchman's "large amount of doubt as to the necessity of
mechanical restraint in the treatment of the insane;"
and his firm belief, on the other hand, "that tranquillity and order among the insane are in an
inverse ratio with the amount of violence, mechanical
or moral, which is employed in treating them."

Such, happily, appears to be the conviction at
which nearly all the superintendents of the large

English asylums have arrived, or to which they are approaching; and all perceive, or begin to perceive, what it is one object of the present work to demonstrate, and what Dr. Hitchman has well remarked, that " the compound word non-restraint is a short term to express the absence of all irritation, and to imply the presence of everything that is calculated to soothe the troubled mind into healthfulness and peace."

Proofs accumulate, indeed, every year, that the best principles of treatment now find almost general acceptance. There was for a time no asylum in which such strong demonstrations of dislike to the new system were made as in that at Wakefield; but even there, the coercion-chairs have been at length destroyed, and the medical superintendent, Mr. Alderson, in a report dated January 1, 1856, says :—" No mechanical restraint has been used during the past year, and seclusion has also been considerably diminished."

If, among the events occurring thus, from time to time, in the various asylums of England, and the opinions resulting from them, one proof of the progress of the non-restraint system could be more gratifying to me than another, it would be that afforded by the latest report of the York Retreat. (*Fifty-ninth Report*, 1855.) It was there, as I have already gratefully acknowledged, that the principles of humane and enlightened treatment

were first avowed and practised sixty years ago,
when William Tuke succeeded in founding that
institution; and it is still in Mr. Samuel Tuke's
description of the Retreat that the student may
advantageously study them; whilst in the Retreat
itself he will find them steadily and unostentatiously maintained.   The entire abolition of
mechanical restraints, although spoken of respectfully and kindly by the same benevolent man,
nearly half a century afterward (1841), was
subjected to very careful inquiry and experiment
before it was virtually, although even then scarcely
professedly, adopted by the physician to the
Retreat.   But the eventual establishment of this
system, and the spirit in which it is preserved, are
instructively shown in the following passages of the
late report, made by Dr. Kitching.

" Among the male patients admitted this year,
one has exhibited symptoms of a rather troublesome
nature, one of which consisted in an incessant
endeavour to make his escape.   As he was by trade
a worker in iron, a bench was fitted up to enable
him to work at his own business, and every effort
was made to allay the morbid restlessness with
which he was tormented.   So unceasingly present,
however, was the one idea, and so persevering the
impulse to put it into practice, without regard to
the means employed, or the risk incurred, that no
other way of detaining him appeared left, but to

engage an attendant who should be constantly with him, like his shadow. After a few months, peculiar nervous symptoms made their appearance, which rendered the prosecution of a noisy mechanical employment intolerable to him. For some time this patient has been employed in the fields and gardens, by the side of his attendant, but the propensity remains still in full force. It has the character of a blind impulse, and on the occasions when the attendant's vigilance has been eluded, the ingenuity and labour which had effected the escape were insufficient to contrive the means of evading pursuit.

" The difficulty of such a case suggests the idea of cutting the Gordian knot by imposing some kind of mechanical restraint, which should impede his locomotive powers; and if the duties of the establishment to the patient were limited to the safe custody of his body, recourse to mechanical restraint would have been both justifiable and expedient. But it is not so. We must take the present difficulty, and use it as a glass, through which to look forward to the patient's restoration; and we are then held to the consideration, whether a state of mind evincing all this impulsive restlessness is more likely to be restored by a mechanical impediment to free movement, or by the absence of such restraint, and by occupation at the workman's bench, or in the fields. And if active employment

continued through so many months, and frequently
varied with experiments whether he or his attendant
can run the fastest, together with the application
of all the moral and medical treatment that could
be brought to bear upon the case, has been
insufficient to remove the unfortunate propensity,
is it at all probable that mechanical coercion
would have had a more tranquillising effect? The
presumption is, that either the propensity would
have acquired additional urgency by forced repression, or the disorder would have manifested itself
in a worse form. The tendency to degeneration of
type has been already betrayed, and if, in spite of
all the efforts that have been made, and the expense
that has been incurred, to produce a better result,
the disorder should degenerate into a more
unfavourable form, it will be a consoling reflection
to those who have had the management of it, that
no means have been used which could by any
possibility promote so unfortunate a termination."

The whole manner in which this case was viewed
at the Retreat abounds with useful precepts for
those who are for ever deterred from casting aside
the vile instruments of restraint by mere phantoms
of difficulty. Difficulties must be expected in the
attempt to abolish such inventions, although they
torture and degrade the patients, and vitiate the
whole treatment in the houses in which they are
relied upon ; but the difficulties are such as inge-

nuity, and humanity, and a determination to do without restraints may surmount. In every difficult case, the physician should consider, as the physicians of the Retreat did, that mechanical restraint merely meets the immediate difficulty, and neither shortens its duration nor prevents its recurrence ; that it purchases present ease at the expense of the patient, and, if it prevents his being troublesome, also prevents his being cured. These sentiments, and the practice based upon them, are consistent with the pure and benevolent views which animated the founders of this admirable asylum, and who, in originally naming it the *Retreat*, meant that it should be "a place in which the unhappy might obtain a refuge ; a quiet haven, in which the shattered bark might find the means of reparation or of safety."

Acquainted very accurately with the effects of the new system, as shown to them by repeated official inspections, the Commissioners in Lunacy, whose gradual approval and careful support of the new system has been already mentioned, put their seal on these general views of what asylums ought to be, and expressed themselves in terms so decisive, and yet so temperate, in their Eighth Report, which has been more than once referred to, as to make an impression on every reasonable mind. Their conviction will not, indeed, prove less influential for having been slowly arrived at.

" As the general result," they say, " which may fairly be deduced from a careful examination and review of the whole body of information thus collected, we feel ourselves warranted in stating that the disuse of instrumental restraint, as unnecessary and injurious to the patients, is practically the rule in nearly all the public institutions in the kingdom, and generally, also, in the best conducted private asylums, even those where the ' non-restraint system,' as an abstract principle, admitting of no deviation or exception, has not in terms been adopted.

" For ourselves, we have long been convinced, and have steadily acted on the conviction, that the possibility of dispensing with mechanical coercion in the management of the insane is, in a vast majority of cases, a mere question of expense, and that its continued or systematic use in the asylums and licensed houses where it still prevails, must in a great measure be ascribed to their want of suitable space and accommodations, their defective structural arrangements, or their not possessing an adequate staff of properly qualified attendants, and frequently to all these causes combined."—*Eighth Report.* 1853. P. 42.

Such is the deliberate judgment pronounced by the Commissioners in Lunacy. It is supported by the opinions of nearly all the physicians experienced in public asylums, and by many of those engaged in private establishments.   In a few more years, it is to be hoped, and it is even most probable, that there will not be raised against it one dissentient voice.

In the preceding record of the progressive practice of non-restraint in the English asylums, reference has chiefly been made to the large public institutions ; but the example set in them has forced some degree of reform into every institution for insane persons, however private.   Even in work-houses, although still deficient in the proper means of treating the many recent cases almost unavoidably sent to them, the principles of treatment are better understood than formerly, so that the number of furious cases brought into the county asylums is probably less than it used to be.   The old method of at once, and indiscriminately, fastening down every troublesome patient, made many frantic who are now preserved from that dreadful aggravation of their malady, and preserved by the kindness and judgment of the medical officers of parish unions. The very great improvement in private asylums has been mainly promoted by the indefatigable industry of the Commissioners in Lunacy during the last ten years; but some of the improvement, it is but just to say, has been spontaneous on the part of the proprietors of the most respectable of such establishments, men of high character and education, and not without a considerable sacrifice of money. It is yet to be regretted that licenses cannot in all cases be restricted to persons so qualified and disposed; and that the most specious appearances, including prompt and wonderful unfastenings and dressings of the astonished patients, are too successfully employed to make the inspection of the Commissioners futile. As too many of the private asylums are still deficient in the means of non-restraint, and either superintended or visited by medical men who have taken no pains to acquaint themselves with the practice of large asylums, I have never ventured to say that mechanical restraints can be wholly abolished in them. It occasions, therefore, no great surprise to find that the managers of only thirty-seven private asylums, out of eighty-four from which returns were made to the Commissioners, had contrived to conduct their houses without mechanical restraints when the Eighth Report was published. There is too much reason to fear that, in the forty-four other private asylums from which no returns were made, the discreet silence proves the preservation of most of the old abuses. The excuses offered, in the answers from some of the private establishments, for their adherence to the use of restraints are such as would be considered unsatisfactory, and even frivolous, in any public asylum in which the system of non-restraint is understood. They consist, for the most part, of the old arguments as to the calming influence of restraints, and the economy of using them.   By precisely the same arguments the employment of chains was anciently defended.

It is deserving of observation that restraints appear chiefly to be resorted to in the smaller private asylums: and that the patients are in many such establishments extremely neglected I have had most convincing proofs ; some of which have been furnished in houses of considerable pretension. The most sensible of the patients in these ill-conducted places are, indeed, well treated, and are sometimes taught to praise the proprietor, or, to use the language of one of them to me, " to show how happy they are."   They are seen by their friends in the best apartments, and addressed in terms of endearment ; whilst the rest, those who are occasionally excited and abusive, those who are imbecile, or apathetic and silent, are kept in wretched abandonment.   Some of these unfortunate beings, when removed to a better asylum, are found to have been in a sort of half-starved state for a length of time, and the cleanliness of the person quite neglected ; the very hair being matted together for want of washing and combing.   In such abandonment they cannot improve; and yet in many of these cases recovery is found to be possible under proper treatment.   I have invariably

found that the use of restraints in private establishments was associated with these neglects; and,
as far as my own observation has extended, I have
never known *all* the patients properly attended to
so long as even a few of them were habitually
subjected to mechanical coercion. Restraints and
neglect may be considered as synonymous; for
restraints are merely a general substitute for the
thousand attentions required by troublesome
patients. The obstinate adherence to a system so
objectionable creates, doubtless, the strongest argument against private asylums, and in favour of
their suppression. But it is too certain that, if
there were no private asylums, the richer patients
would be generally secluded, shut up in upper
stories, or in small habitations; and under the care
of mere attendants. Happily, also, there are
private asylums in which the richer patients enjoy
all those advantages which are found so favourable
to recovery in county asylums for the poor, combined with all the more extensive means applicable
to the insane of the most cultivated classes of
society. The exceptions, it is to be hoped, will
gradually cease to exist.

In the mean time, it is surely incumbent on
all practitioners among whose patients a case of
insanity occurs, to give careful consideration to the
character of the asylum fixed upon for a temporary
residence; and neither to imagine the selection
of small importance, nor to be deceived by con-

temptuous references on the part of the proprietors of small private establishments to the liberal system professed in the large asylums of England. The artful deception practised by those who merely trade in lunatics is sometimes difficult to detect; but the degree of medical attention likely to be afforded to the patient may be estimated by the character and experience of the medical men attached to these houses. Exclusion from all parts of the establishment except the tawdry reception-room is generally a suspicious circumstance; and some conclusions may be drawn from the appearance, dress, and manners of the patients, and perhaps more from the apparent character of the attendants. I have, however, known deception carried on so skilfully—appearances of unusual comfort displayed to the visitor of an hour, combined with such a system of perpetual tyranny, with such an absence of liberty of exercise and recreation, such mean and scanty and half-famishing diet, and such general severity and neglect—as to lead me to think that there is no real security except in the character of the proprietors. These important faults can seldom be detected by the Commissioners, or by anybody; and the patients are often afraid to speak; and, not being always to be relied upon, are seldom believed when they do speak. There are, however, private asylums, and, happily, not a few, where the candour and openness manifested to visitors is unmistakeable; and where the apartments, the attendants, the general air of the house, and the cheerful manners of the majority of the patients, are such as to relieve the mind of a patient's friends from the oppressive idea that such places must of necessity be gloomy and comfortless. It seems extraordinary that a physician in general practice can ever consign one of his patients to any private asylum without some preliminary inquiry of this kind; and it is still more to be regretted that so few practitioners avail themselves of the opportunity of visiting the county asylums nearest to them; where, by witnessing what it is practicable to do for the comfort and cure of the poorest lunatics, they would be able to form an opinion as to the care and attention demanded in any private case. There are hundreds of practitioners, in London alone, who have never had the curiosity to see the interior of a well-conducted asylum; although by so doing they might partly supply a great deficiency in their medical experience, and qualify themselves for the better disposing of the insane among their own patients.

I have long been of opinion that, except in a very few counties, the provincial inspections of asylums by the visiting magistrates are extremely inefficient. The periods of their visitations are generally conjectured without difficulty, and even the day of their intended inspection is not unfrequently known beforehand. The owners of the private asylums are, in many instances, their neighbours or friends. If a resolute justice of the peace resolves to look closely into the arrangements of the asylums near him, and insists upon reforms in dismal chambers and dark staircases, he becomes the object of bitter animadversion and the extremest dislike. The generality of country gentlemen and clergymen shrink from such unpopularity; and it has therefore seldom happened that any amendment in provincial asylums has taken place in consequence of the representations or suggestions of the visiting magistrates; and that nearly all improvements have sprung from the urgent and even repeated remonstrances of the Commissioners. This circumstance seems to point to the benefit that might arise from an extension of the number of Lunacy Commissioners, by which more frequent inspections of the provincial asylums, or a more efficient supervision, might be made by persons wholly independent of local influences. Not only would more authority then be exercised over the private asylums in the provinces, but over the provincial borough hospitals, and other institutions, into which improvements are slowly and reluctantly admitted; and still further extended, to solitary dwellings in which it is to be feared there are, in many an unfrequented district, single patients, who may be said to be rather hidden than protected. Some greater protection might also thus be thrown over patients in residences less remote from towns than the lonely farm-houses alluded to; for the greatest existing evils still incidental to the treatment of insane patients, and even the greatest abuses of mechanical restraint, are to be met with in private lodgings, and in detached villas, the supposed advantages of which often cause them to be selected by the friends of patients who can afford to pay for perpetual seclusion. In many of these, patients of the higher ranks, and of the richer classes, are, I am perfectly convinced, more unfavourably placed, and subjected to more neglect, more mechanical restraint, more dull seclusion, and more indignities of all kinds, than any pauper in the realm. In by far the greater number of these instances which have come under my own observation, the attendants especially undertaking the care of these patients of superior rank have been idle, and presuming, and not particularly sober; more anxious for their own ease than for the comfort of the patient, and always raising objections to the due exercise or any troublesome indulgence of those under their charge; and at the same time exacting preposterous remuneration, and demanding wine, brandy, and other extras, which the friends of the patients, anxious to keep such guardians in good humour, were almost afraid to refuse. Not unfrequently, these attendants have received a bad education in some of our large asylums; where a confederacy usually exists among them, by which their malpractices are often long undiscovered. Being dismissed in succession from different services, they inscribe their names on a list in some advertising office, or some association professing to supply attendants, and still pursue their business for a time very successfully. Female attendants, supplied from such places to private families in sudden emergencies, are often no better qualified; having run nearly through the same career. There are exceptions, both among male and female attendants, and most respectable and valuable persons; but every physician who practises in this department of medicine knows how seldom they are to be met with. Unfortunately, too many families of aristocratic pretensions set the chief value on the effectual concealment of those of their relatives who happen to be mentally afflicted; and even estimate attendants in proportion to their presumption, or their assumption of authority over the patient. They would, indeed, in some instances, rather allow a relative to perish in an upper story of a country mansion, or in a cottage-prison, than have him recognised as insane upon the widest heath where he could enjoy liberty and air.

And thus, too often, the worst effects are produced in recent attacks of mental disorder, in which the early treatment decides the issue of the case. When a patient recovers from an attack in which

the early treatment has principally consisted of
being fastened down in bed, and left at the discretion of attendants for many days or weeks, the
impression made upon the patient's mind is always
unfavourable, either by leaving recollections of
what has been done which cause frequent paroxysms
of angry excitement, or by inducing reflections of a
melancholy nature ; and in either case retarding the
cure, and for a time rendering the convalescence
doubtful.   The scenes to be witnessed, indeed,
in such cases, when first visited by a physician
accustomed to the treatment of insane persons
without restraints, are scarcely credible.   Two,
three, or more able-bodied attendants are found
unable to control one gentleman-patient, unless he
is confined in a strait-waistcoat, and has his feet
fastened.   They allow him no exercise ; and if he
moves they throw themselves upon him.   His
condition becomes beyond all expression wretched ;
and I believe death has often been the consequence
of such treatment.   Delicate young women
affected with mania are tied to the bed, or half-
smothered by servant-women and men, or fastened
down by sheets twisted into the shape of cables,
and tightly bound round the body and round the
bed.   In this miserable condition cleanliness is
neglected, and the patient suffers from heat and
thirst, and becomes exhausted by vain struggles.
The patient becomes rapidly emaciated, and per-

fectly frantic. Nothing can allay the irritation created by the useless crowd, by the disorder of the room, and the closeness of the atmosphere, and all the horrors which in the course of a few dreadful days have been needlessly accumulated about the chamber of a patient labouring under an excited brain, and whose malady all these things do but increase. But in these unhappy cases the friends still often oppose measures of a different kind, preferring the absolute secresy thrown over the malady before all sensible considerations. Their prejudices and weakness find support in the arguments or insinuations of attendants, who are glad to be relieved from trouble, and who commonly neglect to provide against any danger, except by debarring the patient from muscular movement as much as possible, and as long as possible. If, happily, such cases are transferred to the care of attendants who have been taught not to rely upon, or even to have recourse to, restraints, the alteration effected in a day or two is such as to make it difficult to believe that the patient is the same person seen before. If the patient is removed from home to a tranquil asylum, the change is greater still. At home the patient is, perhaps, the cause of indescribable confusion: all domestic regularity is interrupted, the servants speak in whispers, the neighbours avoid the house. Days and nights are passed in anxiety or terror. But the patient who has unconsciously caused all this disturbance, becomes, when taken to an asylum conducted on good principles, quite an altered person; disturbing nobody, and behaving peaceably, and even seeming happy among new associates, and in scenes unconnected with the real or imaginary griefs of the home so lately quitted. Such sudden improvement certainly almost exceeds belief; but the instances of it are not even rare. Every physician conversant with practice in cases of insanity must have witnessed these almost marvellous metamorphoses many times.

I have often observed with pleasure that a kind attendant on a private patient generally becomes regarded in the light of a friend, to whose protection the patient, secretly conscious of mental infirmity, feels himself indebted, and to whose judgment he appeals in all the little affairs of each day. Too often, the attendant's previous training, and sometimes the habits of the establishment from which he is sent, unfit him for acquiring the confidence, and regardless of obtaining the good opinion, of the patient, over whom he assumes an intolerable authority, insisting on instant obedience, either in matters of small importance or such as might more advantageously be deferred—forcing his victim, for example, to take food when he has no desire for it, or medicine when he is disinclined to do so, or to walk out when he would rather rest;

instead of waiting for more favourable times for all these things. Quarrels thus ensue; high words, blows, a tremendous struggle, injury to both parties, and the investment of the vanquished patient in a strait-waistcoat or leg-locks, with which the attendant is provided; from which time the patient becomes more irascible, less manageable, and sometimes, by the severe nervous agitation, further advanced in malady.

The evils arising from the generally indifferent character of attendants, and from their deficiency as to the resources they ought to possess, are so great that few things would benefit the insane more than devising some remedy for them. This might partly be found in an improved government of our larger asylums, where the attendants are frequently appointed without proper testimonials, and without any regard to their temper and disposition. In visiting public asylums in various parts of the country, I have several times recognised attendants whom I knew to have been dismissed from other asylums for negligence or cruelty. The mere appearance of too many of them is so repulsive as to have an unfavourable effect on all patients. For the irregularities into which most of them fall, excuses may be found in the peculiar nature of their duties; in the obstinacy and violence they meet with in their patients; and the want of sufficient occupation or change; and

in their own want of resources to fill up vacant
intervals, and to make up for the absence of
common domestic enjoyments, of regular work,
and of ordinary companionship. Their want of
education, generally, in an age when so much is
done for the education of all classes, is quite
extraordinary.

It would not be difficult to make arrangements
in public asylums for training respectable young
men and women for the duties of attendants; and
for furnishing those only with testimonials of good
conduct who really deserve them. Such arrangements, however, are not consistent with the present
defective organization of some of these institutions;
in which the authority of the officers is so divided
that attendants dismissed for cruelty to the patients
may find some officer in the asylum who recom-
mends them for several good qualities, and who
chooses to conceal the worst. But if due care
were taken to educate the attendants in all the
parts of their various duties, and to inspire them
with a just ambition to manage their patients
through an exercise of the affections and the
reason, rather than by any dread of their authority,
they would afterward be found most useful in
private asylums or in families. Compliance with
the desire of the Commissioners—entertained and
expressed by them ten years since—that when an
attendant is dismissed or leaves any situation for

misconduct, the cause of such change should be reported to them, would also produce good effects ; and it would be still better if, such opportunities of instruction being given as I have mentioned, no attendants were allowed to take charge of insane persons in private houses without a diploma of their fitness for the office, either gained by services in a public asylum, or upon undoubted testimony from the proprietors of private houses, or from private families in which they have been engaged ; such diploma being authenticated by the Commissioners. If a register of attendants could be kept at the office of the Commissioners, and each attendant supplied with a ticket of registry, to facilitate reference, an additional protection would be afforded to the public. Their age, experience, and state of education, should be noted in the register, and particular qualifications; as their possession of any knowledge of amusing games, or of music—accomplishments of considerable value in relieving the tedious hours spent by private patients under their charge. The governors of the large asylums would do an essential service to their deserving attendants, and through them to innumerable insane patients in private asylums, or not in asylums at all, by affording them the means of improving their education; not in mere grammar and penmanship, but the acquisition of branches of knowledge too little cultivated, yet pleasant and in some degree easy of acquirement ; as, for instance, some branches of natural history; and also in music and drawing ; and in some mechanical arts, as turning ; and in other occupations, as gardening. By the possession of these advantages, which they have seldom had any opportunity of acquiring, they would become more cheerful and more companionable when attending patients of education.

Sometimes, whilst revising these pages, the impression derived from recording so many instances of the improved treatment of the insane has made me doubt whether the details into which I had entered, and certain repetitions which were unavoidable, might not even be pronounced unnecessary ; the ameliorations recommended having already taken place, and all the advocated reforms being apparently established and secured. But, even on the eve of publication (July, 1856), I find, in the Tenth Report of the Commissioners in Lunacy to the Lord Chancellor, and no less in some passing events of great interest in one of the largest asylums near London, fresh incitement to continue the advocacy of principles which are still received with unwillingness and delay, or imperfectly understood, in several establishments, and ever prone to be departed from in others. The state of the larger asylums and hospitals for the insane in England appears, from this latest report of the Commissioners, to be still in every year improving : and no allusion is, of course, made to a recent proof of the introduction into one of the asylums just alluded to of practices so severe, in cases of refractoriness, as to confound the heterogeneous ideas of treatment and punishment— practices favourably regarded in one-half of the building, and, as will often happen when there is no medical chief, dissented from in the other half. As long as the government of the large asylums is so constituted, uniformity of practice will not exist in the different parts of any asylum; and opposite methods, sometimes the mere offspring of contradiction, or of petty rivalry, must prevail; and the most objectionable modes of treatment find partial favour.

But it is in the private asylums that the old abuses are still the most obstinately adhered to. Those readers who have been at all interested in the brief history of the altered treatment of the insane, advancing gradually now for more than sixty years, will find, with surprise, in the report just printed, that in one private asylum, close to a large manufacturing town, the asylum containing thirty-four patients, none of them paupers, five of the male patients are lodged in an out-building; that the bedding is insufficient, and the beds are hard and knotty; that four of the female patients, most probably accustomed to the decencies of comfortable life, dine in a room without a table, and that whilst at their meals they are wholly unattended.   In another private asylum, near one of our richest cities, an asylum containing thirty patients, none of them paupers, the premises are dilapidated, the furniture and the bedding deficient, the galleries and bedrooms very cold, the floor of the rooms wet and dirty, the water-closets without water, and the privies filthy.   The state of this particular house seems to have been the subject of frequent animadversion, but improvement has not yet followed.   In another private institution, near a fashionable watering-place, in which there are only three patients, one of them, a young lady, was found in the kitchen, tied down to a chair by a rope, her dress dirty, and her hands fastened to a leather belt.   The same young lady was at night fastened to her bedstead by a strap. What was called seclusion was practised in this case by putting the patient in some small place near the stables, and without a window; where, also, she often slept at night.   In another asylum, containing twenty-four private patients, the Commissioners found, in December, 1855, so many defects as to cause them to advise that, unless very marked improvements were adopted, the license should not be renewed.   Cold and poorly furnished rooms, insufficient bedding, moss-covered garden walks, untrodden by the patients, who were restricted for the most part to a small dull yard, were among the characteristics of this place, where, as might be expected, mechanical restraint was also frequently resorted to. In some other private asylums, where paupers are still received, the accommodations continue to be still worse. There is every reason to conclude that the proprietors of some or all of the houses in which the Commissioners have noted these deficiencies and faults are persons to whom licenses have been improperly granted by the local magistrates. Such an abuse of the power of licensing is far from being uncommon; and every instance of it is an unfairness towards those who have taken pains to qualify themselves for taking care of patients before seeking a legal qualification to do so. The results are assuredly such as ought not to be known in the present day. It is to be hoped that all the proprietors of private houses into whose hands this Tenth Report may fall, will turn to the list of county asylums and hospitals, forming part of Appendix A, and reflect on the contrast presented by the arrangements yet considered necessary in so many of their houses, and those adopted in at least forty public institutions, where the patients, about fourteen thousand in number, are provided with every comfort, and never subjected to any form of mechanical restraint. If, with some of them, no higher consideration weighs, and no sense of responsibility except at the quarter-sessions, they ought to reflect that the patience of the public has its limits; and that if, in their penurious and ill-managed establishments, they have been unable to provide for ladies and gentlemen any of the advantages now enjoyed by a large majority of insane paupers for seventeen years, their establishments must be suppressed.   The only regret such a measure would occasion would arise from the indiscriminate loss or ruin in which better asylums might then be involved; for there are many which are so well conducted as to leave scarcely anything to be desired; and if such retreats did not exist for the richer and higher classes, many of them would be exposed to serious risk of private confinement, where their treatment would be concealed from every protecting eye.

Upon the whole, however, in this country, there is nothing left of the old system calculated to discourage the expectation not only that the manner of treating insane persons without ever having recourse to restraints will soon be so far understood and appreciated as to be almost universally adopted, but that the old deceptions and abuses in private asylums and private houses must soon exist no more. The accomplishments and general character of the candidates for appointments in our county asylums; the admirable reports issuing every year from those institutions, recording every variety of improvement and progress; the clinical instruction already given in some of them; the generous desire evinced by the majority of the county magistrates to make proper provision for the insane poor; together with the continual and even minute attention given by the Commissioners in Lunacy to all that passes in both public and private asylums, are among the circumstances justifying very sanguine hopes of the conservation and extension of all good principles of asylum management. Frequent and liberal discussion of the various subjects connected with lunacy and with asylums has also lately been productive of benefits which will go on increasing. The varied contents of the "Psychological Journal" established by Dr. Forbes Winslow, and conducted with great talent and energy, have attracted the attention of many general as well as professional readers to considerations more or less connected with the welfare of the insane. Still more recently, the formation of an Association of the medical officers of asylums, has been an indication of their sincere wish to profit by the experience of each other, and to unite in advancing an elevated branch of pathology and therapeutics; for which the establishment of " The Asylum Journal" now so ably edited by Dr. Bucknill, affords every facility, by the diffusion of information, interesting and instructive to all readers whose duties, whether medical, or magisterial, or general, have any relation to insane persons. The general character of our public asylums, conducted chiefly by members of that association, is already honourable to us as a nation; furnishes an example which is "a globe of precepts;" justifying the expectation that no false economy, and no delusive theories, will ever lead to the abandonment of the non-restraint system, which comprehends and binds together all the details of sound principle and humane practice. The system, as now established, will form no unimportant chapter in the history of medicine in relation to disorders of the mind. It has been carried into practical effect in an intellectual and practical age, unostentatiously, gradually, and carefully; and is, I trust, destined to endure as long as science continues to be pursued with a love of truth and a regard for the welfare of man.

No longer residing in the Hanwell asylum, and no longer superintending it, or even visiting it, I continue to live within view of the building, and its familiar trees and grounds. The sound of the bell that announces the hour of the patients' dinner still gives me pleasure, because I know that it summons the poorest creature there to a comfortable, well-prepared, and sufficient meal; and the tone of the chapel bell, coming across the narrow valley of the Brent, still reminds me, morning and evening, of the well-remembered and mingled congregation of the afflicted, and who are then assembling, humble yet hopeful, and not forgotten, and not spiritually deserted. The contemplation of the vast exterior of the wings of the asylum still deepens the happy impression, that through all that extent of ward and gallery, kindness and watchfulness ever reign. And when my thoughts are transferred from this, my home-asylum, with its thousand patients, to nearly forty large public institutions for the insane in this great country, in which are more than 13,000 patients, to whom similar comforts are afforded, and throughout which the same system prevails, I find a reward for any share I have had in promoting these things, beyond my deserving ; a consolation in years of comparative inactivity, and a happiness far overbalancing the pains and troubles incidental to my life, as to that of all mortal men.

PART VI.

PROGRESS OF THE NEW SYSTEM ON THE CONTINENT.

WHILST the changes now described have been making in the English asylums, it is to be confessed and lamented, that the treatment of the insane without mechanical restraints has found little favour on the continent of Europe. All the old and most objectionable forms of mechanical coercion have, it is true, been banished from the Parisian asylums, of which the general condition excites the admiration of every visitor. But the strait-waistcoat is still accounted an indispensable auxiliary to the general treatment. This seems so little consistent with the liberal views detailed in the Reports of the Asylums of the Department of La Seine, already alluded to (part 1, page 6), that it can scarcely be doubted that in a few more years the *camisole* will follow the long abolished chains into disuse and oblivion. In the first and second of those reports, the question of restraints is argued ably and candidly; and it is truly enough asserted that except in England their total abolition has received no countenance. The arguments adduced against the non-restraint system are chiefly taken from the Report of the Commissioners published in 1844, containing views very different from those since zealously and efficiently maintained by them.

Among the most influential opponents of the non-restraint system in Paris I number some of my most valued friends; and it is with great diffidence that I put myself into anything like a controversial attitude in relation to them. But I know them to be humane, and lovers of truth, and do not fear their misapprehension of any of my expressions. It is, indeed, the high character and wide authority of those eminent persons which renders their views of importance.

A private communication from the celebrated Dr. Nasse, of Bonn, to Dr. Weber, of London, who obligingly wrote to him for me, and a recent publication by Dr. Daniel Tuke, of the York Retreat, show that the German, Prussian, Austrian, and some of the Dutch physicians continue to use precisely the same arguments. I believe, however, that in Holland I may mention Dr. Everts and Dr. Van Leeuwen, and at Copenhagen, Dr. Hübertz, as standing nearly, if not quite, alone,

among continental physicians, in favour of entire
non-restraint ; and they are almost the only
continental physicians known to me who have
had sufficiently ample opportunities of acquainting
themselves personally with the treatment pursued
at Hanwell, and in other English asylums, and to
which the name of non-restraint system has been
given. On the return of Dr. Everts and Dr. Van
Leeuwen to Holland, they adopted the system in
the asylum of Meerenberg, near Haerlem ; but
under some disadvantages, opposed to the perfection
of the experiment.* With respect to all the other
continental physicians, it is to be observed, that
although unanimous in expressing disapprobation
of the non-restraint system, no one of them has
given it a trial. Their want of observation of the
system in England would indeed make any trial on
their part incomplete. Many foreign physicians
have accompanied me through the wards, most of
them arguing rather than observing ; and some,
I fear, have been conducted through them by
officers regardless of the effect produced, and
negligent of required explanations. Arguments,
however, so unexpectedly used as those revived in
the French report, and so extensively disseminated,
call, at least, for a respectful, although brief,
consideration. We must forget, for a time, that

* The Prize Essay of the Society for Improving the Condition of
the Insane. 1854. By Daniel H. Tuke, M.D., Assistant Medical
Officer to the York Retreat. (Page 44.)

Pinel left on record that when lunatics were relieved from chains in which they had been bound for many years they became less dangerous to approach; that their days and their nights, heretofore agitated and noisy, became tranquil. We must set aside the testimony of Esquirol, who, with forty years' experience, tells us that after the relinquishment of severities in asylums, many accidents diminished in frequency ; and who regarded all severe measures as so objectionable as to advise that they should be deputed to inferior ministers, and not apparently participated in by the physician, whose office they would degrade, and whose influence they would vitiate. Let us, then, examine the arguments employed on the continent.

1. It is asserted that *it is necessary to possess a prompt and great authority over the patient, to induce him to submit to salutary regulations.*

Conceding this, the question is, whether this authority is so certainly and so safely obtained by means of fear, as by gaining the confidence of the patient. The question is fully answered by all experience in favour of the gentler method.

2. *Although influence is for the most part obtained by mildness and persuasion, there are cases in which the physician must show his power.*

No principle seems in reality to be more erroneous. Even when the physician of an asylum must exert his power, he should avoid a mere display of it; by which display the patient who is the subject of it will always be offended, and will long remember the offence. Besides, the argument implies that violence must be subdued by violence; and such was the ancient rule. Modern science regards violence in an insane person as a symptom of a disordered brain; and the physician, refraining from exasperating this disordered condition, tries to allay it; and, discarding all idea of mere subjugation, provides for the protection of the patient, and applies himself to the cure of the distempered state.

3. *The temporary and judicious use of mechanical restraints generally produces tranquillity during the day, and repose at night.*

My own observation in relation to these supposed effects of restraints leads me to look upon this assertion as one of those which are too heedlessly made, chiefly by physicians not resident in asylums, who, visiting the asylum only occasionally, and not daily, rely upon the observation of others respecting the result of measures prescribed by them. Ordering restraints to be imposed at one morning visit, and seeing no more of the patient that day, or in the night, or even the next day, they are not really acquainted with the immediate effect of the restraint. To the same cause may be ascribed the long prevalence of many therapeutic errors, as in relation to

the effects of venesection, counter-irritation, mercurial medicines, and sedatives. Certainly, as
respects restraints, my own observation of the
results of their imposition, and of their discontinuance, which I felt it for a long time most important
to watch, both by repeated visits during the same
day, and often also in the night, when constantly
residing in the Hanwell Asylum, justifies me in
giving the most positive and unqualified contradiction to the assertion of the tranquillising effects of
any kind of coercion. In some of the wards at
Hanwell where violence by day and noise by night
formerly prevailed more than in any other part of
the asylum, the disuse of restraints seemed completely to alter the character of the patients ; and
now, for many years, violence and noise, by day or
night, have been exceptions to the general condition
of the house. In public institutions, and in private
practice, I have scarcely ever seen a patient in
restraint who was quite safely to be approached :
anger has almost always been superadded to
maniacal excitement ; reproaches and curses have
been employed as substitutes for the restricted
muscular movements ; and revengeful advantage has
often been taken of any incautious visitor or
attendant, so as to make a relaxation of severity
very difficult. Many, closely fastened down to the
bed, would spit at those who came near them, or
bite them severely. Some, more malignant and

more powerful, obtained the means of inflicting long-meditated injuries on those having the charge of them. Almost every inconvenience of this kind disappears, or is transient in its duration, where seclusion, alternated with exercise (as it always ought to be), is substituted for mechanical coercion. The increased tranquillity of an asylum, by day and by night, is, in fact, one of the most remarkable results of discontinuing such coercion.

4. *Mechanical restraint is a surer means than any kind of superintendence of preventing the patient from being hurtful to himself or others.*

It must here be observed that if a patient's hands are fastened by handcuffs, he can still both strike and kick; and that he can run violently and knock people down by his mere weight and impetus. Therefore, positively to prevent injury to others, the mechanical restraint must be extended; the feet must be fastened as well as the hands, and so closely that the patient can scarcely move about at all; or he must be completely fastened down. And, as regards security to the patient himself, if security from suicide is meant, the experience of every asylum has proved that there is no such security in restraints; and that suicides have become rarer since restraints were discontinued. A patient in restraints becomes also hurtful to himself by unavoidable uncleanliness; and is, moreover, helpless when attacked, and more liable to be thrown down and injured.

The arrangements of an asylum must be very defective in which no kind of security or protection exists except restraints.   In such an asylum the attendants are few in number, inefficient, and permitted to be habitually careless.   Such was always the case in the days of restraints.   Patients were allowed to quarrel, and no pains were taken to pacify them.   To violent words violent actions succeeded, and fights ensued; and then the attendants rushed passionately on the combatants, putting them indiscriminately in restraints, and dragging them into dark rooms, by way of punishment. There the angry patients remained until the next morning; no record of their seclusion being kept, and little attention or none paid to their condition. I merely mention what I often saw in my early experience at Hanwell, and what the wanton use of restraints unavoidably led to.   All these evils of treatment hang together by a chain which the abolition of restraints breaks at once.   That broken, the number and character of the attendants becomes properly attended to; vigilant supervision is exercised; kindness proves more powerful than leather or iron; the patients are occupied and amused—walked with, talked with, and made cheerful; they are kept clean and comfortable; both physical and mental causes of irritation are as much as possible kept from them ; quarrels become rare, and are never prolonged ; and, among other good results, the disposition to suicide disappears. All these effects, and all this protection, were never produced by restraints.

5. *In large asylums it is necessary to employ attendants who are not always to be trusted, and whose patience is often severely tried, so that their best security is to put the violent patients in restraint.*
This is surely a dangerous apology for cruelty. In small asylums, as well as in large, the patience of the attendants is often severely tried ; but in neither is it necessary to employ attendants who are not always to be trusted. To employ them knowing that they are not to be trusted, and to allow them to protect themselves by putting their patients in restraints, is to consign the patients to systematic brutality. Bad-tempered attendants are always in the most danger in asylums, and most naturally look for safety to the use of restraints ; and, becoming heedless of better means of control, have frequent struggles with the patients, in which somebody is always hurt. The violent patients, thus treated, become still more dangerous; all the other patients are disturbed or alarmed ; suspicion, deception, and revenge, become common in all the wards ; and thus, the confidence of the unhappy patients never being won, their general improvement is most cruelly obstructed.

6. *In most circumstances, restraint by the strait-waistcoat irritates and exhausts the patient much less than the personal struggle required to force him into his cell, where, left free in his movements for several hours, he may hurt himself, or commit suicide.*

To this the answer is, that no personal or prolonged struggle is required to put a patient into a quiet room, if it is properly done by a sufficient number of attendants; and that it is not difficult to exclude all means of suicide, or of injury to a patient, in a padded room: whereas a strait-waistcoat cannot be put on a violent maniac by any number of attendants without a somewhat long personal struggle ; and when put on it is not really a security against suicide.

7. *In small asylums, the system of non-restraint requires a staff of attendants out of all proportion to the number of patients.*

This is the favourite argument of the proprietors of many small and wretched asylums which ought to be suppressed. For patients in wealthy circumstances, several private asylums now exist in which the number of attendants nearly equals the number of patients; and there are excellent asylums for all patients in tolerably good circumstances in which the attendants are in the proportion of one to three or four of the patients. For the insane of the middle classes, generally, and of the educated classes in narrow or indigent circumstances, especially, there are now asylums combining all the resources of public institutions with most or all of the comforts of the best private asylums :—such are those of Northampton; of Coton Hill, near Stafford; of Cheadle, near Manchester; and the fine establishment superintended by Dr. Browne, near Dumfries, called the Crichton Institution. So that in Great Britain, at least, this argument is entirely without force.

8. *Coercion, practised with mildness and pru-dence, at least permits the patient to take exercise in the open air ; whilst, by any other system, the patient is in a state of seclusion, which is only restraint under another name, and in another form; and may be followed with moral results more unfortunate than those produced by mechanical restraints.*

This objection to the disuse of restraints is wholly based on the erroneous supposition that all violent patients are in perpetual seclusion. But in our English asylums no patient is, or ought to be, deprived of daily exercise who is able to walk; even although, after such exercise, seclusion may still be necessary for the rest of that day: and, this being attended to, seclusion becomes every day less and less necessary. During the daily

A A

exercise, as no restraints impede the movements of the patient, every muscle is left to its free or even to its irregular and eccentric action; and such action is often remedial. A patient walking in a strait - waistcoat exercises half of his muscles only; he is cabined, and cribbed, and uneasy, and is a spectacle of distress to the other patients. The unfortunate moral results are as imaginary as the state of entire seclusion is in which they are supposed to supervene.

After repeated consideration of all the foregoing arguments, which were first employed in England twelve years since, and are thus resuscitated abroad, I cannot avoid a feeling of surprise on finding them employed to justify a system of treatment which in the course of those years has been all but universally abandoned in this country. The most reasonable conclusion to be drawn from it is, that the accomplished physicians of the Continent, who appeal to these arguments, cannot have examined, or even witnessed, the non - restraint system in actual operation ; and that they are also too slightly impressed with the innumerable abuses and horrors of the old system—the system which was purely based upon the principle that the insane must be controlled by force, and governed by fear alone. If these recollections existed in sufficient force, means of control, which are really at variance with all the principles of French practice as much

as of those of the English, would not be honoured
by such advocacy. But are they really unacquainted
with the past, or forgetful of it ? It may seem
superfluous, or almost tedious to be once more
referred to them, after what has been said in the
preceding pages ; but yet a general view of the
necessary and inevitable sequences of what seems
so simple and plausible a thing as the imposition of
the camisole should make any humane physician
shrink from deserting the path of scientific and moral
treatment for the mere vulgarity of a constraining
and torturing dress. Not to revert to the days
when flogging and horsewhipping were practised
and praised, they cannot have forgotten that in the
old asylums, too much resembling those from which
sprung up the arguments they now condescend to
employ, every object continued, even so late as
fifteen years ago, indicative of captivity, and suggestive of gloom; that the windows were still
closely barred with iron, or half blocked up with
iron panes as substitutes for glass ; that the tables
and benches were as clumsy as those in a felon's
cell, and were even fixed to the floor, whilst
many of the bedsteads or cribs were made of
massive wrought iron as if nothing was safe
from desperate violence ; that in every gallery,
at that time, the visitor was met by a powerful
surly male attendant, or an ill-dressed nurse,
who seemed to have lost all habitual expres-

sion of kindness ; that each of these guardians
had a press full of all the curious instruments of
restraint—fetters of all kinds, collars and straps
resembling harness, iron handcuffs, leather leg-
locks, chains, and gags—all of which they could
employ at their pleasure ; that every crib had
arrangements at the head and foot, and on each
side, for fastening down the patient at will ;
that rows of coercion - chairs were to be seen,
in which patients who had been fastened to the
cribs all night, were fastened on a kind of close-
stool all day ; with results painful and furious,
which even Dr. Jacobi, who lauds these inventions,
has graphically described.

In the very airing-courts of those old asylums,
which were, indeed, but dismal yards, there were
strong rings in the walls, sometimes still to be seen,
although no longer used, hanging above the miserable benches where then the patients sat chained,
in sunshine or rain, in heat or cold, for hours
together ; no attendant near them, to speak to
them, to give them water to drink, or to guard
them from the violence of the other patients.
Food, in those restraint days, was given to the
patients in the most careless manner ; and several
of them swallowed it all at once. There were often
neither knives nor forks ; table-cloths had not
been imagined ; and the plates were iron. In what
manner they slept at night, on what beds, with

what clothing, who can now describe? Yet there was as stout a defence made for all this system, of which these things were but a part, as if it had comprehended every advantage. No measure of hostility was thought unjustifiable towards those who tried to put an end to it. Indeed, the officers of asylums were accustomed to rely on rude and overpowering means alone, and could not comprehend how they could be dispensed with; so that their resistance to all novelties was earnest. The attendants were few in number, inefficient, relying wholly on mechanical restraint to meet every evil and inconvenience; and destitute of all other resources; so that every relaxation of discipline seemed to them perilous. Amusements, occupation, instruction, secular and religious, were laughed at, in those old institutions, as the suggestions of philanthropic craziness. There was no relief or pleasure for the eye, or ear, or any sense or faculty. Whilst there was everything calculated to distress the disordered mind, there was nothing to promote its recovery.

I do not imagine that any advocate for the use of mechanical restraints wishes to see all this restored; nor is it to be believed that in the present day the superintendent of any asylum would be permitted to restore such abuses: but the continental advocates for restraints may be assured that in whatever asylum mechanical restraint is avowedly often

resorted to, many of the evils and neglects of which
I have spoken do also still actually exist, and must
exist; which might, indeed, if necessary, be illustrated by very recent examples, taken from the
institutions of our own country.

Mechanical restraint spares so much trouble,
it renders the management of the insane so compen-
dious, it makes a number of expensive attendants so
superfluous, that it is difficult to resist the tendency
of the mind to preserve the habit of making use of
it.   When established, as a part of the system,
in any asylum, it always became by degrees the
predominating part.   Its progress was uniform,
certain, inevitable.   The recently received patient
was   irritable,   abusive,   menacing;   or   he   was
dejected, silent, and reported to be suicidal.   The
argument being that violence is best restrained
and suicide best prevented by mechanical coercion
—the argument still cited and employed—it was at
once resorted to.   From the melancholic patient,
whose melancholy was increased by it, the cautious
superintendent   never   removed   it.   The   more
irritable patient, indignant on finding that a single
attendant tried to manacle him by main force,
struck the attendant; and his restraints were made
additionally severe.   The sleeves, or the strait-
waistcoat, or the muff, were resorted to.   Then
the patient walked or ran about violently, and
gave passing kicks to other patients, or the

doors. His feet were consequently next secured in hobbles; or, more convenient still, the attendant dragged him to a bed and fastened him down, hand and foot, and head, to repose as best he might. The patient's only resource then was to be noisy: no restraints could control the tongue; so, excepting an occasional attempt to stop his breath with a pillow, the attendant allowed him to rave as long as he liked; and there he remained, day and night, frantic, noisy, hungry, thirsty, and half poisoned with dirt. He filled the building with curses; and the other poor patients were truly "with terrors and with clamours compassed round." Perhaps he became silent, and was pronounced tranquil: if not, restraints were still accumulated upon him, until, in time, he lay quite subdued, the triumph of the restraint system. Soon, however, some strength returned; he shouted, swore, raved, blasphemed, and the terrified spectator saw him heated, flushed, feverish, foaming at the mouth, perfectly maddened. What effect all this had upon the irritable brain may be imagined: irritation was of course aggravated into more intensity, sub-inflammation often followed, and the results were organic and irremediable changes. If the violence subsided, it was succeeded by sullenness and refusal of food; and then the last and finishing resource of the restraint system was resorted to: the tube of the stomach-pump was forced down his throat; there

was a fearful struggle, and sometimes the struggle
was fatal. Thus, if the patient had yet any chances
of relief, they arose only out of the various proba-
bilities of death. He lost strength; ulcerations
supervened; his feet mortified; and he died in
restraints. And after death alone, I know,
partly from personal observation, and partly from
unquestionable authority, proofs of violence were
too often found, to which the unprotected patient
had been subjected during life. Fractured ribs,
and fatal lesions of internal organs, violence done
to the bladder by the rude introduction of the
catheter, rupture of the œsophagus and trachea
by the tube of the stomach-pump, have been among
these proofs; and these have exclusively been found
in the old asylums in which restraints were
employed, or in those where, although resort to
restraints was not permitted, some officer or other
was still secretly attached to the system to which
they belonged.

I know that the abolition of restraints from our
English public asylums must make the most faithful
description of things existing previous to that
abolition seem exaggerated. Many of the excesses
of restraint, also, are avoided, or very carefully
concealed, even in asylums in which the principle of
restraint is still cherished. But wherever restraints
are employed, the tendency to these excesses
remains; and if, unhappily, the general use of

restraints should, in the capricious revolutions of medical opinion, again be established, however modified or palliated by discreet description, all security for the proper treatment of insane patients will be taken away : one abuse will follow another, all kinds of neglect will gradually be practised, and the slow re-introduction of the most detestable parts of the old treatment will be inevitable. Assuredly the good physicians of Paris would start with abhorrence from countenancing the possibility of such abuses being revived or prolonged. Yet there is many a lunatic, in various countries on the Continent, still pining in a wretched cell, or secured by restraints, in consequence of the extreme influence deservedly exercised by French opinion in all matters of medical science and practice. But with a recollection of all those evils which, however now condemned, were once universal, and found apologists everywhere, surely every physician in every country should try every resource before constituting himself the advocate of mechanical restraints. Certainly no physician can with propriety defend them who has not taken the trouble to make himself acquainted with the details of the more humane system which he condemns. And there is nothing more certain than that the events of one single month in any asylum where restraints are not used would be sufficient to satisfy any candid observer that the removal of restraints was in all cases followed by advantage; and that the health of the body, and consequently of the mind, was most strikingly promoted by the various humane substitutes for it. No one, after such experience, would consent to undermine a system diffusing such wide and general benefits through asylums, for the sake of meeting a few trifling difficulties in separate cases.

In the foreign asylums, where there is so much to be admired, it must yet be admitted that there are practices tolerated, and even common, which too forcibly illustrate the impossibility already asserted of combining a complete system of general kindness and attention with the habitual use of the camisole. No one can doubt that the physicians of the Continent are animated by the strongest desire to alleviate, in every respect, the condition of the insane; and there is a painful inconsistency in the spectacle presented in their asylums, of patients coerced in restraint-chairs for no better reason than that they are restless, or mischievous, or merely feeble and troublesome. Where but in the Continental asylums should we now behold a dozen pails of cold water thrown over an unresisting and shuddering man because he is indisposed to work? Where else should we at this period find an example of a wretched creature fastened down in a crib for many successive years? Or where else shall we now find the douche employed merely as a punishment, and a column of water allowed again and again to descend on the naked head, or to be propelled with cruel force on the face of a helpless victim fixed to a board so contrived as to receive it, and present it to this outrage—and all perhaps because the patient, afflicted in mind, has been careless or indolent, or has even persisted in cherishing some harmless delusion?* Where but in some large asylum where the camisole and coercion-chair are cherished shall we find such a scene as that described by Dr. Van Leeuwen, and which is probably still exhibited—nearly forty dirty and paralytic patients in a ward, without an attendant; half of them without either trowsers or drawers, some tied down on their backs, seven in strait waistcoats, many sitting on comfortless benches; and all the wretched furniture, and the very ground, permeated with horrid odours? These things, I repeat, are an almost unavoidable part of the system in which mechanical restraints are relied upon. They are among things inseparable from habitual recourse to coercion; and those excellent men who defend mechanical restraints so warmly are unconsciously defending every cruel abuse to which a poor defenceless lunatic can be exposed.

Most deeply is it to be regretted that so eminent a physician as Jacobi should give his formal sanction to the use of coercion-chairs—instruments of

* Dr. Daniel H. Tuke's Essay, pp. 39, 41, 46.

restraint so galling that he is compelled to recom-
mend their being of the strongest workmanship, on
the ground of its being "incredible with what
violence many maniacal patients will convulse themselves" when so coerced.* The same great authority
speaks in praise of a "coercive basket" in which
the patient is laced to a narrow sack and pillow. In
M. Guislain's Medical Letters on Italy, there are representations of several ingenious methods of bodily
restraint in use on the Continent, and well known,
it appears, in Germany. By one of these, a strait-
waistcoat is put on, and then fastened, as well as
the patient, to a mattress fixed up against the wall.
The sleeves of the waistcoat are fastened on each
side of the body, crossed over. The legs are provided for by being placed within a kind of drum,
preventing flexion of the knees. This is described
as being in use at Aversa. In this way patients
are sometimes kept safe and fast for seven or eight
days together. M. Guislain scarcely approves of
these things; but still, generally judicious as he
is, he was disposed to import from Venice another
device for keeping a refractory patient's legs and
arms quiet. By this invention, the lower part of
the patient's body is put under a ticken stretched
on a frame across a crib. The chest, arms, neck

---

* On the Construction and Management of Hospitals for the
Insane, &c. By Dr. Maximilian Jacobi. Translated by John
Hitching; with Introductory Observations, &c. By Samuel Tuke.
London: 1841. Page 177.

and head are on the outside of the ticken; but the arms are extended at full length, and fastened down at the wrists and elbows.   One cannot wonder that the Venice asylum, where M. Guislain saw these things, abounded with cries and restless movements; and that the spectacle of the female patients fastened to their beds, in the upper story, their waxen cheeks, black hair, bare bosoms, wild laughter, and loud imprecations, *stupified* him, although accustomed to the ordinary scenes witnessed in asylums.*   The more, indeed, that such perversions of ingenuity are substituted for kindness and for the thousand attentions required by afflicted maniacs, the more must the asylums containing them assume " the air of hell."

Such barbarous methods must in every year, in every country in the world, become more rare, until they disappear altogether, as the heavy chains and harness have disappeared from the asylums of England.   It is the more surprising to find physicians so highly distinguished as those engaged in the special practice of insanity in Paris, and attached to their fine establishments for every form of mental infirmity, and others not less able and accomplished in Germany, whose names are known all over the world, adhering to any of the old abuses, or suffering even a remnant of them to disfigure their asylums, and to throw discredit on the

* Lettres Médicales sur L'Italie, &c., p. 249.

times. Every page of the French Reports, already so often mentioned, contains illustrations of the care extended to the insane in the large asylums of the French capital; and especially of the anxiety to render the buildings, by every scientific appliance, wholesome and cheerful.* The principles which guide and animate the good *alienist* physicians of Paris are evidently identical with those zealously cherished by the non-restraint physicians of England; and these principles will assuredly lead to perfect conformity of practice. We owe an ancient and great debt to the French in relation to the insane; and it is to be hoped that they will not think it an unworthy condescension to borrow something from us in return.

There is a disadvantage to contend with, forming some excuse for the resort to restraints in the Continental asylums, in the imperfect adaptation of the buildings to the purpose for which they are intended. But the chief excuse or explanation is, the want of an intimate acquaintance with the system pursued in England; a deficiency which it is partly the object of the present work to supply; and which a patient observation of the daily routine of many of our large English asylums, by efficient

---

* The task of drawing up these valuable Reports devolved, I believe, chiefly on my much esteemed friend M. Battel, one of the Directors of the Civil Hospitals. They furnish an admirable model for such documents.

medical men deputed from Paris for the purpose, would probably remove. The observation of such deputies should, however, be systematic, and consecutive for many weeks, under the guidance of superintendents who would earnestly assist or direct their inquiries.

One of the best accounts of the English asylums published on the Continent within the last few years, and which also contains the fairest view of the non-restraint system, is that of Dr. Henri Curchod, of Lausanne; who appears to have visited England and Scotland with a sincere wish to obtain accurate information respecting asylums, and to have been very diligent in collecting it from good sources.[*] A very candid and liberal report was also made to the Prefect of la Seine Inférieure in 1853, by M. Deboutteville, the director of the asylum of St. Yon, at Rouen, and M. Mérielle, the chief physician of that establishment. These gentlemen were deputed, with the architect of the Département, to visit the principal asylums in England, preparatory to the preparation of plans for rebuilding the asylum of St. Yon. Their remarks on the construction of our asylums, on ventilation, warming, and all other details—and also on our medical and moral treatment—were

* De L'Aliénation Mentale et des Établissements destinés aux Aliénés dans la Grande-Bretagne. Par Henri Curchod, Docteur en Médecine. Lausanne, 1845.

minute and exact; the few inaccuracies committed being partly to be ascribed to their having to visit seven different asylums, in as many different counties, in the short space of ten days; and partly to their omitting to visit the Hanwell asylum altogether. Of course these gentlemen, although well fitted for the task confided to them, and remarkably free from prejudices, had no time nor opportunity to study a system which provides for exigencies deemed by them decisive as to the necessity for the occasional use of the strait-waistcoat. Their opinions, however, are so courteously expressed, and their general views so liberal, as to show that the difference, after all, between the English and French practice is not, as I have already said, based on opposite principles; and that uniformity of method will before long prevail in both countries. Nothing would more effectually promote this than an arrangement by which a certain number of young medical men, deputed from Paris, could reside for a month or more in some of our best asylums, so as to be able to observe the daily occurrences and various resources of those institutions. Or if the design of our English association of superintendents could be so extended as to admit foreign associates, and to induce them to attend the annual meetings, an interchange of visits with the French and German physicians might be established with excellent results to all countries.

CONCLUSION.

I now bring this book to a close. I have endeavoured to show what was the nature of the old method of treatment of the insane, and to describe the more comprehensive character of the new method now generally practised in this country. Although many reasons induced me to detail the early steps of this treatment at Hanwell, I have not forgotten that I might be regarded as a partial witness, and have, therefore, adduced the testimony of other physicians, whose authority and whose candour are beyond question, and who are attached to other asylums, where they have watched the progress made in the same direction. I have not attempted to conceal the objections which lately prevailed in England, and continue to be entertained by many physicians of eminence in other countries, against the entire abolition of mechanical restraints, nor the difficulties which they believe to be necessarily consequent on such abolition; but I trust I have shown that these objections are not formidable, or even sound; and that all the supposed difficulties may be avoided.

To one subject I must still revert, which has

long weighed upon my mind ; namely, the imperfect
government and organization of all asylums for the
insane in which the functions and duties of the
medical officers are not regarded as of the first
importance—asylums in which, if the patients are
numerous, the medical officers are few in number,
and without the direction of a chief physician.
In such asylums the committees supply, or ought
to supply, the office of superintendent or governor.
Committees vary so much in character, and are
sometimes, even, so remarkably modified for a time
by the predominating influence of some one individual, that what may be said with perfect truth
and justice of a committee in one year, may be
inapplicable to it in the next. This changeful
character has, however, great disadvantages as
respects the discipline of an asylum, even when
the majority of such governing body consists of
men of liberal education. Usually the committees
are greatly occupied with financial and economical
regulations, in which they are experienced and
skilful. They are generally not so well qualified to
make regulations affecting the tranquillity of the
patients, or the comfort of the attendants and
officers. Alterations which appear to them expedient, and, especially, formal arrangements copied
from the usages of prisons, are often found by the
physician to produce annoyance to the patients, by
reminding them that they are merely looked upon

as lunatics. The physician's opinion respecting such details is probably, however, considered fanciful. At the ordinary meetings of the committee, the reports made by the medical officers scarcely receive the attention which their general importance should command, and they are sometimes treated as superfluous. A system, essentially vicious, by which reports are required from all the officers, encourages counter-reports and contradictions, which are mischievous. Not only is information sought for by the committees from the chaplain, the steward, and farm bailiff, which may be necessary, but the assistant medical officers, and the dispenser or apothecary, and the matron, all make reports, and generally all make medical reports; in which they are permitted to comment on the chief physician's report-book, if there is a chief physician. Thus arise divisions and dissensions, which usually weaken the credit, and disturb the peace of mind of them all. According to a well-ordered plan of government, all the officers should report to a chief physician, and he alone, in ordinary circumstances, to the committee. One effect of these multiplied report-books is the introduction of unnecessary matter, and sometimes of trivial and foolish details, leading to the loss of much time in mere desultory conversation, unproductive of any good consequences whatever. A worse result is that sometimes, under sudden impulse, produced by a rash observation in some one or other of the minor reports, strong determinations are arrived at by the committee, without reference to the physician, even when affecting some question which ought to be referred to him. He receives an official notification of these decrees with astonishment and mortification; but, fortunately, the resolutions passed so unreflectingly are often forgotten as soon as the impulse which occasioned them passes away, and are never acted upon. Yet many inconsistencies originate in this manner; the government of the house retains no fixed character, and no officer knows how he may be affected by some random regulation on the next committee day. In short, instead of possessing the stability and rational liberty arising from the consistent government of one chief, acting according to something resembling a settled constitution maintained by a committee, asylums thus regulated are a sort of miserable republics, where nothing is constant but inconstancy, and nobody feels secure. And yet on the general state of mind of the officers, and even on their being made comfortable and content, and allowed to lead a peaceful life, the happiness of the patients largely depends.

Except the great task of educating young persons, and especially those whose birth and station will early enable them to exercise an influence on society as legislators, there is perhaps

no office that requires higher qualifications of mind
and heart than that of the directors or governors
of institutions for the care and cure of infirm or
disordered minds. But this truth has received
so little attention as to appear scarcely more than
a paradox to those who have never given five
minutes' consideration to the importance of the
duties undertaken by all who accept such an office.
The office is at present assumed by gentlemen who,
however honourable and kind, are commonly only
selected, in the larger counties near London or
any large town, from those who live nearest to
the asylum, or those whose activity and habits
of business, acquired in professions or trade, cause
them to be perpetually on some county committee
or other, where they prove in common matters
eminently useful. In the less populous provinces,
and when the asylum is in an agricultural district,
the committees usually consist of country gentlemen; and of them it may be truly said, that if, in
some instances, they are scarcely qualified for such
high duty, they amply make up for any defects by
a generous confidence in the physician, and by
an habitual liberality in their general arrangements.
In the committees of the metropolitan asylums we
find, of course, few country gentlemen; but also
few men of scientific or literary acquirement; and
scarcely ever anyone who has studied the human
character with any view more elevated than that of

worldly gain. They are generally able men, acute, and often benevolent; but not physiologists. Yet, whoever knows the insane, knows that no one is qualified to legislate for them, or to make even trifling regulations for them, still less to govern them, who has not been long accustomed to consider how the human being is influenced by various circumstances, physical and moral, acting on the bodily health, on the senses, on the feelings, or on the understanding. Such duties cannot be properly performed, or even safely undertaken, by men who are ignorant of all the agencies of a physical nature, in health and in sickness, which modify the manifestations of the mind. Governors of institutions for the insane should possess something even beyond all this:—a tone of mind softened, disciplined, and tempered in the world ; not excited by vulgar prosperity, but possessed of such natural sensibility as to ensure sympathy with those whose malady is encompassed with sorrows.

This training is seldom acquired in the ambitious walks of public life, or in the office of business, or in the routine of retail trading; and yet the committees of asylums, to which each of these busy worldly departments contributes, have almost an irresponsible power in immense establishments intended to be places of relief for all the shades of disordered mind.

In this country, so many auspicious circumstances

surround those born in all the classes above indi-
gence, that virtues are developed where their
growth could scarcely be expected; and often, with
the utmost exercise of shrewdness and keenness in
transactions entered into merely for profit, there is
conjoined a generosity which, in such conjunction,
is so unexpected as to appear almost romantic.
My grateful recollection of several of the members
of the Hanwell committee, most of whom death
has now removed, will never die. From the
ranks of merchants and others, educated almost
exclusively to cultivate the means of accumulating
wealth, I have seen men step forth, animated with
every benevolent feeling, and anxious to encourage
whatever was really generous and good. These
excellent men have felt all the disadvantage of acting
with men of a different mould; for it too frequently
happens that in proportion to the unfitness for the
exercise of such authority, there is a fondness for the
display of it, and a kind of vain pleasure in thwarting
the views of the medical officers, and indulging
the unwonted privilege of possessing power over
gentlemen who, except in point of money and
the accidental relation in which they are placed
to them in the asylum, are really their superiors.
When it unfortunately happens that persons of
this last description are either the most numerous
or the most active of the committee, the situation
of the physician becomes painful; suggestions

founded on reasons deduced from his professional study and observation, are slighted, or not even comprehended; and alterations are continually made at variance with all the principles which he wishes to preserve.

Considering the various education of men of different professions and ranks, none would seem so likely to be fitted by their diversified studies, and by the practical application of them to the preservation of the health of men and women, to undertake the mental, physical, and moral government of lunatics and lunatic asylums, as medical men.   Their various knowledge; the attention they must have given to the functions of human beings, separately, and in their several relations; their practised observation of the effects of bodily diseases; their acquaintance with all ranks of society; their constant intimacy with the modifications of both physical and mental phenomena in all the accidents of life; and the very nature of their daily occupations, by which the best human feelings and sympathies are almost necessarily called into exercise, must generally be supposed to impart qualifications to them which are rarely possessed to the same extent by men in any of the other walks of life.   Among the medical superintendents of asylums appointed within the last sixteen years, and particularly since the dawn of what may be termed the mental government of the insane, it would not be difficult to name several who illustrate these pretensions in a very high degree. It is happy for such superintending physicians when they act under the gentle and enlightened control of a committee or board chiefly composed of persons of liberal education and of benevolent tendencies; before whom they can confidently lay the suggestions which some incident in the wards, or some observation in the grounds, may have originated, and on which they have carefully reflected. If they oppose some architectural or other fancy of the committee, they can state their reasons for it, without fear of being misunderstood; and they acquire a reliance on the governing body which prevents their ever being deterred from proposing anything that is really good for the patients; a consideration which they know to be always paramount in the committee, and which excludes meaner considerations from their minds; considerations based on vanity, or a desire for popularity, or on a narrow adherence to economy. Without the encouragement thus afforded to myself at Hanwell, much that has been spoken of in the preceding pages would never have been possible, and some of the most important features of the modern treatment might perhaps not yet have been developed, or put in practice. Still, it can scarcely be supposed that, with an experience of ever-changing committees during fourteen years, I was always so fortunate. In all asylums, there must be periods in which the majority of the members of the committee are unimpressed with the necessity of refraining from giving needless disturbance to officers whose minds, if vexed and fretted, can scarcely be beneficially exerted over the minds of the patients. Some there must occasionally be, on all committees, who do not comprehend that their duties are those of general guardians of the patients; and that their wishes, even when well-directed, can only be carried into effect by able officers, to whom the anxious and agitating practical duties of the asylum must be confided; and who should there-fore, if possible, be allowed to possess their own minds in quiet. Noisy committee-days ruffle the minds of all. The board becomes quarrelsome. The officers are each irritated—perhaps insulted—in turn; and the very patients catch the disturb-ance. Above all, the heart of the superior officer of the asylum must be discomposed and saddened, when he knows, that after such a tempest, there remain for days visible proofs in all the wards of discomfort, distrust, and agitation; and that even the patients, who are always acquainted with such occurrences—taught by some morbid quickness in their acutely sensitive organizations—comment upon them, and sometimes in words from which committees might learn discretion, if not wisdom.

My personal interest in such matters has ceased. The wildest resolutions of committees can afflict me no more. But, knowing too well what rash experiments may be made by committees, and how dexterously all responsibility may be avoided, even when the comfort of a large asylum, and the discipline of the house, and the very health of the patients, are endangered by inconsiderate changes, I cannot avoid some allusion to such things, nor dismiss from my mind all anxiety about them, nor refrain from recording my opinion, founded on long observation, that the proper treatment, and the welfare, and happiness, of the insane is insecure under governing bodies constituted as those of asylums now generally are. Full security might, however, be given to the public, and every advantage to the insane surely preserved, if the control of asylums was always entrusted to intelligent superintending physicians, acting under the general inspection of a board or committee qualified for such superintendence by a liberal education, and by their habits of mind; who would entertain no apprehension of evil from delegating such full authority to the physician as would leave him at liberty to carry out comprehensive plans, according to principles admitted and approved by them; and at the same time possessed of authority empowering him to enforce conformity to his measures among all the other officers. Thus, and thus only, I believe, might be established and maintained a consistent plan of asylum government; advantageous and humane in relation to the patients; encouraging to all the officers of such establishments ; and just to the community at large.

London: Printed by Smith, Elder & Co., 15, Old Bailey.

Milton Keynes UK
Ingram Content Group UK Ltd.
UKHW041521181024
449640UK00009B/115